MW01012822

ACU-CAT
A GUIDE TO FELINE ACUPRESSURE

Nancy A. Zidonis
Amy Snow

Foreword
Jane Bicks, DVM

Illustrations
Carla Stroh

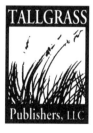

TALLGRASS
Publishers, LLC

Published By: Tallgrass Publishers, LLC
                     1175 South Ogden St
                     Denver, CO   80210-1710

Cover Design: Catherine Connors

Graphic Design   Christine Peterson

Copyright: ©2000 by Tallgrass Publishers, LLC
                     Denver, CO

Library of Congress Catalog Number In progress
ISBN 0-9645982-5-6
        1. Cats   2. Cats – Alternative Treatment   3. Cats – Health

1st Edition 2000
Printed in the United States of America

FOREWORD

For me, and many of the other 55 million cat owners in the US, a cat is very special. While Amy Snow and Nancy Zidonis discuss their physical attributes that help to determine some of their complex behavior plus the success and enjoyment of acupressure on these exceptional animals, let me take a moment to reflect upon their extraordinary sensibilities.

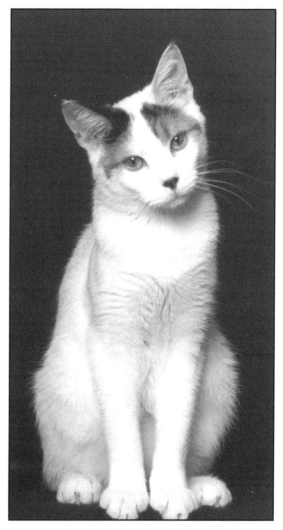

I was always a dog person at heart, until I found a sick little kitten on the streets of Brooklyn. The kitten had distemper and every veterinarian that I went to in Brooklyn strongly suggested euthanasia since antibiotics would never cure this raging deadly disease. I finally found a semi-retired veterinarian who prescribed droppers full of goat milk, honey, bee pollen and anything else a pharmacy student would want to add for immune support. Interestingly, he also suggested that I rub the kitten in various places to stimulate his desire to live and of course give him as much love as I could. Every morning before going to school, during my breaks and in the evening I fed the kitten and rubbed his little body concentrating on the parts he seemed to like the best. Eventually we won the battle and Toshi became part of my soul, graduating with me from veterinary school and living a few years past that. In retrospect I have to thank that old time veterinarian for his prescription of nutritional therapy and whether he knew it or not, acupressure.

Since Toshi, there have been other cats in my life. They share my sorrows, and my happiness. They just have a way of nudging themselves into my spirit, soul and life. They can be stoic animals and keep illness to themselves. Although cats are considered independent, an owner must look at his cat and its daily habits to identify a problem before it gets out of hand. If you take the time to observe your cat, you will notice little things from time to time: stiffness, runny eyes, lethargy, lack of appetite, excessive hairballs, etc. While these are not causes to run to the family veterinarian, it is the owner's responsibility to do something to give their cats relief, just as we would for a child. That is where acupressure can become part of responsible animal ownership. While there are situations in which acupressure cannot replace a veterinarian visit, it certainly behooves a cat owner to learn the techniques in Zidonis and Snow's book.

I believe that veterinarians should study this ancient art – to return to the days when healing was about mind, spirit and body. We need to know how to make our cats more comfortable in our offices and during home visits by applying acupressure. The time has come to integrate traditional medicine with alternative medicine. Once we do that, we will truly be serving our feline family members.

– Dr. Jane Bicks,
Nationally Renown Veterinarian, Author and TV Host.

ACKNOWLEDGEMENTS

We appreciate the love and soft presence of all our felines, past, present and future. We thank them for being in our lives, contributing their spirit, and making this book meaningful.

We are fortunate to have the support and encouragement of Jane Bicks, DVM in creating Acu-Cat. Dr. Jane is a strong proponent of natural healing and has authored four books including *Revolution in Cat Nutrition* and *Dr. Jane's Thirty Days to a Healthier, Happier Cat*. She has appeared as a veterinary expert on numerous radio and television programs and hosted segments of Animal Planet. Dr. Jane heads Trilogy Best Friends, a foundation to promote animal welfare through shelter management and rescue organizations (www.trilogyonline.com).

Carla Stroh contributes her artistic talents as an illustrator. We thank her for the obvious pleasure in drawing animals and adding joy to our books. We greatly appreciate Catherine Connors for her dramatic cover design and relentless good nature. Thanks to Tina Peterson for her text design and sense of humor. And, thank you to our friends: photographer Jan Jones, Sue Green, Donna Tukel, Janet Bayless and all of their feline friends.

A special thank you to our friend and colleague Marie Soderberg for her support through all of our books and her generosity of spirit. We extend a note of gratitude to our families, especially Ann Zidonis, Erica Leah and Haia Rebeccca Pois.

Other books by the authors:
Equine Acupressure: A Working Manual
The Well-Connected-Dog: A Guide to Canine Acupressure

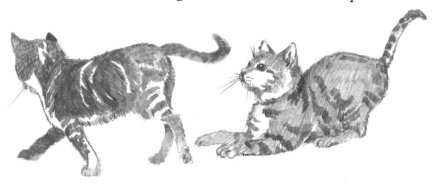

TABLE OF CONTENTS

INTRODUCTION

Cats and Us

Cats have become the most popular companion animal in the world and with good reason. Their small, furry bodies and wily ways are so appealing. Their plaintive meows beckon us to satisfy their needs, yet their natural independent nature relieves us from tending to their every whim. Busy people and those having lots of time to dote over these gentle creatures are happy to live with a cat or two. Cats fit in small places and large spaces. They conform to being indoors or out of doors, romping and tromping. All in all, the domesticated feline is the perfect pet.

Cats have served as efficient mousers since the Egyptians discovered the cats' incredible talent for ridding grain storage bins of vermin. The felines, in turn, were attracted to human communities because of the ready source of prey. Our relationship with cats has been mutually beneficial for the most part. In the medieval period, cats were feared because of their seemingly supernatural powers. They were identified with the devil and viciously destroyed by the thousands. Though this was a pervasive thought at the time, there were still many people who protected cats, knowing that their ability to control the rodent population actually aided humankind.

Cats have earned their keep for hundreds of years. As the twenty-first century gets underway, we have less need for a cat's impressive predatory instincts and more of a need for a softly purring, silky feeling, affectionate companion. The cat has not changed in hundreds of years. Today's felines are just as capable of survival without human intervention as they were in northern Africa. We are imposing our needs on cats and depriving them of their natural environment where they keenly hone their senses for catching fast-moving mice in the dark of night.

Asking cats to live in our world often means that they lose contact with their feline world. Because they must abandon their own way of life to share ours, they are showing signs of stress by demonstrating non-cat-like behavior, developing more frequent immune system diseases and other physical stress conditions. Acupressure offers a way to care for your cat in an entirely different and natural way.

Acupressure is an ancient healing art. This noninvasive, deceptively gentle treatment can profoundly impact both humans and animals. Cats are extremely receptive to acupressure when they need it. Consistently, casework has shown that acupressure can enhance your cat's comfort, emotional stability, and overall health. Specifically, acupressure can:

- Relieve muscle spasms
- Build the cat's immune system
- Enhance mental clarity and calm
- Release natural cortisone to reduce swelling
- Release endorphins necessary for reducing pain
- Resolve injuries more readily by removing toxins and increasing blood supply.

Modern medicine has begun to acknowledge the value of eastern healing modalities. Fortunately, we have the knowledge to make optimal use of both western and eastern approaches and techniques when caring for ourselves and our cats. Given the growing awareness of the benefits of the ancient healing arts, more people are actively participating in their animals' well-being.

Acupressure does not substitute for veterinary medicine or animal chiropractic care. When your cat is ill or injured, we encourage you to consult your medical practitioner and get the assistance needed to resolve the physical injury or disease. Acupressure is an important avenue of treatment that complements western medicine.

We invite you to explore the realm of acupressure to return your cat's loving purrs and willingness to be part of your life. Cats are highly sensitive creatures and understand the language of touch. *Acu-Cat* is a step-by-step guide to acupressure. This book offers you and your cat access to powerful healing and will contribute to deepening your mutual bond.

To bring the benefits of acupressure to you and your cat, we have distilled some of the essence of Traditional Chinese Medicine's (TCM) vast and complex body of knowledge. This book is a journey into the ancient healing arts. We hope this will be an unending adventure for you in learning to heal, share with and care for your cat.

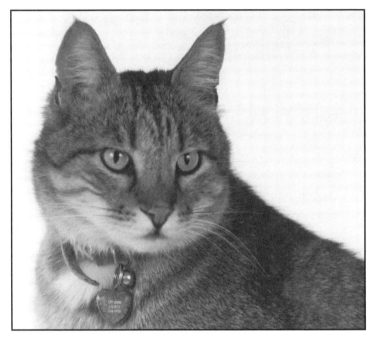

The Cat only grinned when it saw Alice. It looked good-natured, she thought: still it had very long claws and a great many teeth, so she felt that it ought to be treated with respect.

"Cheshire Puss," she began, rather timidly, as she did not at all know whether it would like the name: however, it only grinned a little wider.

"Come, it's pleased so far," thought Alice, and she went on. "Would you tell me, please, which way I ought to go from here?"
"That depends a good deal on where you want to go," said the Cat.
"I don't much care where —" said Alice.
"Then it doesn't matter which way you go," said the Cat.

-Lewis Carroll, Alice In Wonderland

chapter one
Cats Will Be Cats

Our Bond

Cats delight and mystify us. Domesticated cats are distinct from any other animal. We get caught up in their taunting manner, sublime expressions, and soft, silky animal attraction. Ever since cats decided to share their world with us, we have had mixed feelings about them.

The ancient Egyptians considered these sleek, supple, vermin hunters to be deity. While the Egyptians admired the cats' ability to perform their primary task of ridding the grain stores of pests, they also viewed the small North African cat as the connection between the world of darkness and daylight because of their nocturnal prowling habits. The Egyptians believed that the cat goddess, *Bastet,* would protect them from the dangers of the night when humans feel most vulnerable.

The Egyptians were intrigued with the felines' constant contrasts. The cats' soft eyes were contrasted by their relentless hunting instincts. Their seemingly affectionate purring paradoxically opposed their unflappable, stalking nature. When sleeping, the cat appears to be the image of serenity, only to awaken to be a treacherous killer. A rodent is no match for the most benign *Felis Domestica.*

By the Middle Ages, these nocturnal, aloof, solitary creatures had lost their favor. Associated with evil, they were considered devils. In 1484, Pope Innocent

1

decreed cats and cat lovers as subjects of an Inquisition. Cats struck fear into the hearts of medieval Europeans because of the supernatural powers attributed to them at the time. No longer deemed furry god-like charmers, cats were hunted and destroyed by the thousands during the beginning of the Christian era.

Throughout history, whether feared or deified, the felines' redeeming virtue has been their ability to keep the rodent population under control. When the Black Plague spread and threatened to wipe out most of Europe, the 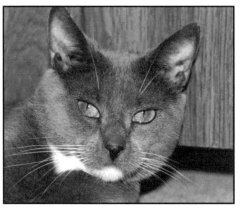 Europeans' aversion to cats diminished. The species survived and cats went on to perform their jobs as efficient mousers and human companions.

Over the course of the next centuries, cats sailed the high seas as royal guests of captains and crews. They traveled to every port and were smuggled ashore and sold for a pretty penny. In the New World, people valued cats so highly that they practically returned to being exalted divinity. In the American West, the pioneers did all they could to get a hold of cats. A kitten could sell for hundreds of dollars, it was so prized. People recognized they won the battle against vermin when cats were at their side.

Today, most people sharing their homes with a cat do not have the same need to rid the houses of rats and mice. In fact, most of us become squeamish when our docile, domesticated kitty brings home a dead baby bird in the spring. We can feed our cats bag after bag of cat food, but our sweet little kitty continues to bat around a half-dead field mouse. Grasshoppers are a summer source of feline antics that also provide them great entertainment.

Thousands of years ago, cats were worshipped as a god. Cats have never forgotten this.
—anonymous

Though there are still many barn cats and other working cats held in high esteem because of their ratting skills, the predominant number of cats live as honored guests in our urban and suburban homes. We have learned to overlook the gifts of shredded birds, hairball regurgitation on our favorite rug, shrieks in mating season and all the other attendant issues of living with a cat.

Feline Protection Resources

There are times that cats need help from their human friends. The big world can be nasty and cruel to these little creatures and they need our protection. The first line of assistance in the case of neglect or abuse is your local animal shelter, animal control, and various cat clubs. There are many volunteer animal rescue groups in most communities as well. If there are no animal protection services in your area, every state government in the United States has an animal welfare office. State governments are responsible for the regulation of pet stores. The United States Department of Agriculture oversees commercial breeding, brokering and distribution of animals including companion animals. Publicly funded resources often have limited staff causing their ability to respond to vary. Resources available are:

The Humane Society of the United States (HSUS) for animal welfare guidance and disaster relief:
Website: www.hsus.org.
General: 202.452.1100
Disaster Services: 301.258.3101

American Society for the Prevention of Cruelty to Animals (ASPCA) for animal welfare references:
Website: www.aspca. org
General: 212.876.7700

United States Department of Agriculture, Animal and Plant Health Inspection Services If you are concerned about the treatment of animals in relation to breeding, brokering, or transporting, please contact:
General Website: www.usda.gov
APHIS Website: www.aphis.usda.gov
General: 301.734.4980

The internet is a valuable resource for other cat rescue and protection organizations and interest groups. Search under "Animal Welfare" or "Cats."

To live as our constant companions, cats have less stimulating lives than if they lived on farms or in the wild. We ask them to adapt to many stressful environments for their species. A city apartment presents little stimulation for a cat's hunting instincts, while it probably exposes our friendly, fuzzy fellows to a host of household and environmental pollutants. In urban settings, cats are apt to be hit by a moving vehicle if left to follow their predatory nature. Suburban cats run the risk of absorbing chemicals from fertilizers when dashing across manicured lawns after squirrels. We offer them quantities of "dead" food for them to consume, which is definitely not their first choice.

We expect our felines to be happy and healthy with all of the trade-offs we provide. Our devotion, cozy homes, relative safety, veterinary care, and abundance of food does not take the place of their nightly stalking of prey, munching on mice, and guarding their own territory. Nothing can substitute for a cat's natural way of life. However, acupressure offers your cat many health benefits to relieve some of the physical and psychological stresses.

Acupressure and Cats

As an ancient eastern healing art, acupressure has been used with animals for at least four thousand years. Though these solitary animals often do not like to be touched, cats are highly attuned to acupressure. Usually, a cat in need of a treatment is cooperative and requires little enticement to receive acupressure work. In our experience, cats respond readily to treatments.

A friend of ours has a middle-aged cat named Stevie who was abused and ignored as a young cat. He developed a serious eye infection that went untreated. Now he suffers from upper respiratory problems and constant drainage from his eyes. When we met Stevie, his coat was patchy-looking with parts that felt stuck together and other areas that were dry and wispy. He looked at the world through small slits and blinked his eyes quickly. His breathing sounded labored with an

Cats are sensual beings, making them willing acupressure subjects.

asthmatic wheeze at the end of each breath. Stevie was obviously very uncomfortable. After his first treatment, we knew he was an excellent candidate for acupressure. Within 24 hours, much of his distress began to abate.

Now Stevie has a rich, lustrous, thick black-and-white coat. There is no swelling around his eyes and he can keep them wide open, although there is continued periodic drainage. He breathes normally, he has lots of energy and is being the cat he was meant to be. Whenever he thinks someone might be willing to give him an acupressure treatment, he backs up with amazing accuracy to the right acupressure point under the person's hand. Cats are sensual beings, making them willing acupressure subjects.

Acupressure is a therapeutic way to actively participate in your cat's health. By learning how to apply acupressure treatments, you can create a close partnership with your cat, which will contribute to years of quality companionship and good health. The relationship you build with your cat through acupressure treatments will enhance his comfort, emotional stability, and overall health. The effects of acupressure have consistently shown the treatment's ability to release endorphins and natural cortisone. These reduce pain and increase blood supply needed for healing.

By combining the ancient eastern healing arts, modern medicine, and loving good sense, you give something special and deeply caring to your cat. We ask our cats to join us in our hectic lives–often not realizing how stressful their lives become. Acupressure gives us a means to mitigate and reduce our cats' stress and tend to their well-being.

When your cat is ill, injured, or experiencing a behavior disorder, you are encouraged to consult your veterinarian, animal chiropractor, or animal behaviorist. To receive the benefits of modern technological advancements, western medicine, psychopharmacology, and animal behavioral sciences are all effective avenues for resolving physical trauma, disease, and severe behavior problems. Acupressure augments western medicine and can alleviate the need for extreme treatments.

The way Dinah washed her children's faces was this: first she held the poor thing down by its ear with one paw, and then with the other paw she rubbed its face all over, the wrong way, beginning at the nose: and just now, as I said, she was hard at work on the white kitten, which was lying quite still and trying to purr – no doubt feeling that it was meant for its good.

–Lewis Carroll, Through the Looking-Glass

In practicing acupressure, as with other Traditional Chinese Medicine (TCM) disciplines, the practitioner considers all aspects of the cat's life and physical characteristics when assessing a cat's condition. We cannot separate a cat's health from his environment, the food he eats, how he spends his time, his amount of daily exercise, his physical traits, response to sound, the look in his eye–everything that characterizes his life specifically. We view the cat and his life as a whole.

The Nature of Cats

Cats are nocturnal, predatory loners who are extremely territorial. If we view feline behavior through the prism of territorial predation and perpetuation of the species, all of a cat's behaviors make sense. Their hours of incessant grooming and long naps during daytime hours prepare them for their nightly hunting expeditions. By being extremely clean, they will not attract any unwanted attention. Their predators or prey will not be able to smell them approaching or hiding. In addition, fastidious grooming leads to fewer parasites and skin infections that would compromise their strength and survival.

Nocturnal Predators

A cat's visual capability is not particularly acute. Cats have a limited ability to see detail but are quick to detect any movement, even in very low light. This makes their eyesight ideal for catching rodents that scurry and feed at night.

Practically every inch of a cat's body is a sensory organ. From the tips of

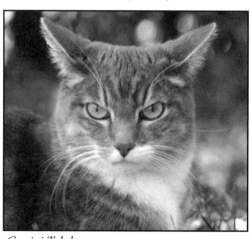

Gemini Tukel

their silky whiskers to the ends of their swishing tails, cats detect lots of sensory cues. The length of their whiskers matches the width of their bodies. If a cat wants to pass through a narrow space or a small hole, their whiskers tell them if they will fit. Rodents tend to hide in small, dark places, whiskers give cats the necessary sensory information to avoid finding themselves stuck in place they can't move or get out.
Cats have extra sensory nerves on the backs of their front legs. When catching prey, they use their front paws and it is important for them to be aware of movement and the condition of their prey. If they were to let go of the small animal too soon, all of their efforts at stalking and chasing would be for naught.

Though their sense of smell goes beyond our own, cats do not use their olfactory senses predominantly to seek out their prey. Mice and other rodents have keen hearing and they would be alerted to a cats' presence if they sniffed the air while stalking the neighborhood.

Aside from the fact that most cats' ears are absolutely adorable and fascinating to watch, cats hear far more than we do. Also, they use their ears to communicate as well. In the wild, it is important to be able to provide visual and auditory cues. When cats flatten their ears, we know it is time to leave them alone, and so do other cats. Most cats prefer not to fight, so flattening the ears is a good sign to move on. If they need to defend themselves, flattening the ears may even protect the ears from being bitten or scratched.

By a minute twitch of the ear, cats gather lots of auditory data. Ears positioned on the top of their heads like external "satellite dishes" function as precise fact finders. Cats can instantly detect the location of a sound plus if it is moving, if it is living, and if it is large or small. An animal who survives on its senses to hunt and catch its prey, while also eluding its own predators, must rely on its auditory perceptions to guide it through the perils of the night.

Since they have been co-habitating with humans, some cats have shifted their life style from nocturnal to diurnal. They spend their days hanging out on the window sill watching the world go by and making cackling sounds at birds in the bushes. Daytime is a good time for extensive grooming, claw sharpening on scratching posts, and taking cat-naps in sunny spots on the living room floor. When food is presented in a bowl, they have less incentive to sleep in preparation for a night of hunting.

Solitary and Territorial by Nature

One way cats lure us into their mystique is by being aloof. The more they act as if they own the house and us–while also being stand-offish–the more we want to snuggle with them. This must be human nature. Conversely feline nature is to be solitary. Since cats had to compete for scarce food resources, they carved out a specific geographic territory and spent their waking hours patrolling and hunting within this domain.

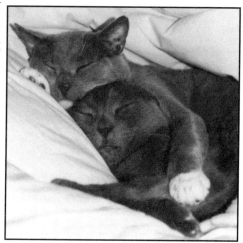

As household pets, cats do not compete for food and they have adapted to smaller territories. Some cats even willingly share space with other cats. As kittens mature into adulthood, they usually stop rolling around in wild furballs and frenetically chasing each other down the hall, only to climb up your favorite curtains. Sometimes it takes a lot of convincing for an instinctually loner-type cat to accept another cat as part of the family. Two females brought up together seem

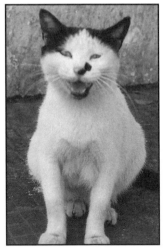

to have the least resistance to living together in adulthood. We have two females who are surprisingly devoted to each other. They groom each other, share food bowls, and curl up together on the sofa during winter afternoons.

Cats territoriality gives rise to their need to mark the boundaries of their spaces. They have their own message system designed to let other cats know whether they are welcome or not. Urinating, spraying and rubbing the scent glands on the sides of their mouths are tell-tale signs that a cat is establishing or reinforcing territorial boundaries. Odors range from very mild to extremely unpleasant. Most of us find ways to mitigate the stronger smells by not challenging our cat's territory, and by keeping his world as stress-free as possible. Although spraying in the house probably cannot be totally avoided, acupressure can increase your cat's overall sense of well-being. This, in turn, may reduce his level of stress and fear.

Cats are so territorial by nature that it is initially stressful for them to move or be adopted into a family with other pets. Acupressure has shown to help cats acclimate to new surroundings and have less trauma when meeting new animals. In Chapter Six, Acupressure Treatments for Specific Conditions, we have included treatments for calming and reduction of fear.

Living Together

Cats have not changed. They still have their basic instincts and habits. By joining our households, they can adapt just so far; we have to adapt the rest of the way. Humans will never totally dominate the *felis domestica*. They will always have their wild side and some behaviors that may cause us distress. A hairball deposited on Aunt Susan's latest crocheting project can create great consternation. Claw marks on a favorite antique chair can bring tears to our eyes. Running to the veterinarian because Darth defended his turf and now has a nasty abscess is no fun.

The best we can do is understand cats as animals we have chosen to be part of our lives. Interpreting a cat's behavior in human terms and feelings leads us the wrong way. For instance, Toby urinates in the basket of fresh laundry and our first thought is that Toby is angry with us. Cats do not have ulterior motives. Toby was simply marking the laundry because it did not smell like his territory, yet it was within his boundaries. Tucker is not bringing you a gift when he drops a dead mouse at the side of your bed in the morning. He knows we will feed him so he does not consume the mouse for nourishment, yet he is compelled to carry out his nocturnal, predatory instincts.

Cats defend their territories. They spray odoriferous signals when feeling threatened or a need to mark their ground. They kill rodents if their mothers taught them how. They prefer freshly killed meat to inert blobs or dry crunchies in a bowl. They yowl during mating season. When left to their own choices, cats are nocturnal. The reality is, the closer we can come to providing the cats' natural way of life, the healthier and happier they will be. Accept the fact that your sweet, affectionate, silky feline friend is a cat in all of his or her splendor.

As parts of our families, cats adapt as best they can and each cat adapts differently. Your handsome Spencer may be completely happy to sleep in sun puddles all day and become the commanding tom in the neighborhood at night. Little Lilly, a delicate Siamese with a reverberating meow, may be too fearful to venture outside at any time of day or night.

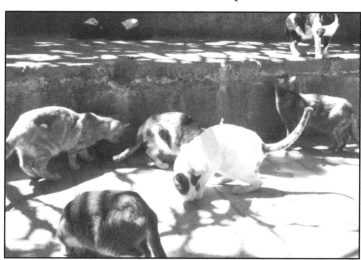

Chellah Cats, Rabat, Morocco

George, a feisty apartment cat, likes to bat every small object around the floor for amusement. Sadie, an elegant Himalayan, cannot imagine having another cat dare to cross the threshold of her house. Cats certainly have their own personalities.

By associating with humans, cats have fallen prey to a host of illnesses and behavior quirks. They have become more prone to diabetes, immune system disorders, skin problems, allergies, heart disease, obesity, urinary tract difficulties, genetic disorders, and other health problems. Cats are often traumatized by frightening things that happen in our urban and suburban environments. While we offer them food and protection from predators unlike their existence in the wild, they still have to contend with other physical and psychological stresses we have given them.

Specific acupressure treatments designed to deal with health and emotional issues will greatly benefit cats. We can contribute to our felines' health and well-being when they accept living under our care and protection. After all, cats and humans share something important. We both need each other. This mutual need is a common denominator. It links us, fostering a bond that makes our destinies inseparable. Cats contribute so much to our lives. Now, through the loving and healing touch of acupressure, we return their gifts.

When the Almighty allotted the means of living, He asked the cat, "From whom do you want to receive your daily bread: the shop keeper, the peasant, or the peddler?"

The cat answered wholeheartedly, "Give me my daily bread from an absent-minded woman who leaves the kitchen door open."

Recorded by Nachum Raphael form Libya, Folktales of Israel, Dov Noy, Editor

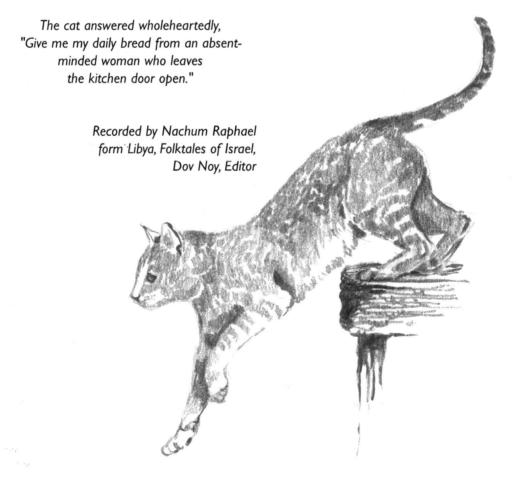

chapter two
Traditional Chinese Medicine

Overview

Cats are the perfect subjects for Traditional Chinese Medicine (TCM) because they are sensitive to the natural balancing of life force energy. Most cats are capable of performing their own healing work. Grooming is a good example of a cat constantly attending to his or her own health needs. When cats groom they not only clean themselves; their scratchy tongue and paws stimulate acupressure points and massage the surface of their skin. Cats know when to eat grasses to clear their internal systems. They know when to exercise, when to meditate, and when to sleep deeply. Once cats trust that we can assist them in having a balanced flow of life, they show us when and how we can help when they need it.

Chapter Two gives a brief overview of TCM and some of the basic concepts underlying acupressure. This will prepare you for your journey into acupressure and the ancient eastern healing arts. Your cat may not understand the words or the concepts, but he knows how good it feels to be in harmony with all that exists.

Acupressure connects you and your cat with thousands of years of natural healing. The source of acupressure lies in Traditional Chinese Medicine. Fully understanding and knowing TCM takes years of in-depth study and practice for it is a highly complex system that is both precise and flexible. Studying TCM is a rich and poetic experience that opens you to new sensations and concepts.

Grasping some of the basic concepts will facilitate your ability to perform acupressure treatments on your cat using the following framework: (1) how and why acupressure can balance your cat's energy (2) the meridian system involved (3) how acupressure works to support your cat's optimum health and joy in life.

TCM treats the mind-body-spirit as a single entity in harmony with nature and the environment.
The Chinese view the body—human or feline—as an intricate and interdependent system in which all aspects of internal life and external environment are intimately intertwined.

TCM treats the mind-body-spirit as a single entity in harmony with nature and the environment. The Chinese view the body—human or feline—as an intricate and interdependent system in which all aspects of internal life and external environment are intimately intertwined. Health occurs when the body-mind-spirit is in a state of harmony and balance with both internal forces and external influences such as cold, wind, or dampness.

TCM developed as a preventive form of treatment. Originally, it was used to maintain the health of livestock, a valuable resource in China. Approximately 4,000 years later, practitioners are still being trained to identify patterns of disharmony, or imbalances, in body energies before physical symptoms of an imbalance can manifest. The TCM practitioner understands that living bodies must be in bioenergetic harmony both internally and with all nature.

Despite the tremendous healing powers of TCM, doctors in ancient China were paid only when their clients remained healthy. If a client became ill, the practitioner was in disgrace and did not expect payment.

In ancient China, the TCM practitioner approached healing from a holistic perspective encompassing many levels. The practitioners medical bag included dietary therapy, exercise, meditation, herbal remedies, massage, physical manipulation, acupuncture, and acupressure. The practitioner observed the patient from many view points, then selected the appropriate healing modalities and assisted the client in integrating these into his lifestyle.

The TCM healing arts share a number of concepts. Following is a list with brief descriptions of the basic tenets common to all. Later, we will explore these concepts in more depth and explain how they relate to the practice of acupressure.

TCM Key Concepts

Chi Energy	The life force energy infused in everything (pronounced Chee).
Yin/Yang	The representation of opposite but complementary qualities that are interdependent and exist in a constant state of dynamic balance.
Meridian System	A one-network system through which Chi energy is carried to all parts of the body.
Acupoints	They are analogous to pools of energy located along the meridians that are used to balance energy.
Eight Guiding Principles	Eight general patterns that assist the TCM practitioner in recognizing the causes of a disharmony in the flow of Chi through the meridian system.
Five Phases of Transformation	A complex conceptual framework that describes five natural phases of transformation. This theory provides an understanding of the "checks and balances" that exist on earth and within living bodies. It identifies the Building, or Creation Cycle along with its counterpart, the Controlling or Breaking-down Cycle. In acupressure, the Five Phases of Transformation are used to indicate how to balance energy and maintain or restore health and well-being.
Balancing Energy	Manipulation of energy to restore harmony and balance.

Chi Energy

The cornerstone of TCM is the life force energy called Chi. In eastern thought, Chi pulses through all life and is present in all of nature. Chi is the basis of everything that exists, including mineral, vegetable, and animal. This vital, dynamic force controls harmony through constant transformation and conversion of matter and energy in a living body and all of the natural world. We impact the total Chi available to us and our cat-friends by the quality of the lifestyles we create. If we exercise, eat good food, breathe clean air, and create a positive environment, we help preserve and create our Chi energy. It is exactly the same for our feline counterparts. Good quality nutrition and natural foods, proper exercise, and a balanced lifestyle help our cats achieve strong and balanced Chi, creating an environment for continuous good health and healing.

Many levels and types of Chi in human and feline bodies are always working in concert. We can identify different forms of Chi by their locations and purposes. However, all the different types of Chi are only one Chi, which merely exhibits itself in different forms.

Western medical practitioners are starting to recognize the value of including TCM in their practices. Research has demonstrated magnetic-type fields that flow along pathways in the body that do not necessarily follow neurological pathways. Conventional western medicine has come to agree that a living body is more than the sum of its biochemical parts. Chi may be invisible, but it is hard to deny it is real whether we call it Chi, "Prana," or magnetic force. Understanding bioenergetic medicine supports biochemical medicine in allowing the body to heal itself. All any medical practitioner can do is assist in creating an environment for healing, the body-mind-spirit creates health.

It is important to note that when TCM refers to an organ such as the lung or spleen, it refers to the entire organ system affected by the organ. That is, when the lung is discussed in TCM terms, it means the lung's function in relation to the whole body. For the purposes of this manual, we discuss only the major forms of Chi and how they relate to the overall well-being of your cat.

Source Chi is given to offspring at conception and is the basis for Kidney Chi. It is stored at the Source Points of each meridian. This Chi is closely related to essence, or Jing, and is the hereditary Chi each animal receives at birth. Source Chi is the foundation of all Yin and Yang energies in a body. Every individual human and cat is born with a fixed amount of life force energy. Source Chi can be depleted by illness, poor nourishment, and an unhealthy environment. Source Chi lessens over time until death.

Through careful breeding practices or natural selection, plus a healthy lifestyle of

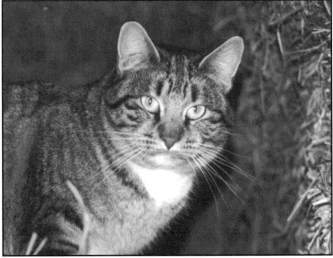
Minu, a healthy barn cat

the queen and male, every kitten starts out with a healthy amount of Source Chi. Since Source Chi is not replenishable, it is up to the cat's human to provide a wholesome diet and healthy, balanced lifestyle throughout the cat's life. Kittens who come into the world with too little Source Chi to sustain them are likely to fall prey to disease.

Chest Chi is extracted from the air we breathe. Lungs inhale clean Chi, transform it for the body's use and exhale stale, spent Chi. This continuous exchange and extraction of Chi keeps the body's physiological processes functioning properly. Exercise adds to the strength of the body's lung capacity. Barn cats and indoor-outdoor cats usually have enough physical exercise and psychological challenges to maintain their own balance of healthy Chest Chi. Unfortunately, indoor cats need far more exercise and environmental stimulation than they are able get each day. All cats thoroughly enjoy being their natural predatory selves whether they are stalking a ball of crumpled paper or a scooting, live mouse. Cats need to breathe clean air while using their lungs and muscles so that Lung Chi optimally circulates throughout their body's.

Since few cats are able to be the hunters they originally were intended to be, people devise new toys for their cat athletes. Apartment cats definitely like environmental enhancements such as multi-level jungle gyms and cat guardians to play toss-the-toy-mouse down the hall. A long stick with feathers dangling from one end can keep both cat and human amused and active. Scratching posts and empty paper bags left on the floor can suffice.

Food Chi, derived from food and drink, is released in the stomach after the digestive process changes food into body nutrients. Food Chi plays a major role in supplementing the types of Chi that are not inborn but can be created during the cat's lifetime. This is why TCM attributes great importance to the quality and quantity of food that nourishes the body's energy.

Unlike dogs, who are "opportunivores," cats are primarily carnivores. Cats must eat meat no matter how much a vegetarian guardian wishes it were not true. Cats have happily and healthfully survived on live food prior to human co-habitation and for hundreds of years after. When cats ingest live rodents, herbivores, they are also consuming the contents of their stomachs. This is how cats originally received the vegetable nutrients necessary to maintain a healthy, natural diet.

Processed cat food is a relatively new human invention. None of the commercial manufacturers really know what a cat's complete nutritional needs are. In fact, we are seeing that many cats fed processed food alone are developing cancers, heart disease, obesity, skin problems, neurological disorders and other diseases not seen in the cat population until recently. We do know cats are perfectly healthy when they eat raw meat, fish, insects, birds, and reptiles with small quantities of well-cooked grains and vegetables. Some veterinarians and nutritionists recommend that meat needs to be 65% to 75% of a cat's diet and the rest vegetables. Feeding a cat human-grade food helps avoid parasites and toxicity.

Commercial cat food manufacturers are not bound by food standards or regulations in most countries. To advertise that their food is "balanced" or "natural" means very little. If you are feeding your cat packaged or canned food, for your cat's benefit we suggest investigating higher quality foods at your local specialty pet store. Also, consider giving your cat raw, natural meats and fish, perhaps blended with a better processed food product. Quite a few cat nutritionists, veterinarians, and top breeders recommend a diet of raw food for excellent growth and health. There are many new cat nutrition books and natural pet publications available to help you learn more about a healthy diet for your cat. Some of these books are listed in the Bibliography section.

Kittens learn what is safe and what is not safe to eat from their mothers. During a kittens formative period, six to sixteen weeks, their mothers bring them food and show them how and what to hunt. This early training is patterned into adulthood, which is why it can be difficult for a cat to change foods even for reasons of better health. It would serve a young kitten well to be exposed to a variety of foods before he or she becomes a "finicky" eater.

A cat's Food Chi will be enhanced by shifting to natural foods just the way we feel better when we eat less fast-food and better home-cooked meals. Our bodies know the difference almost immediately, and

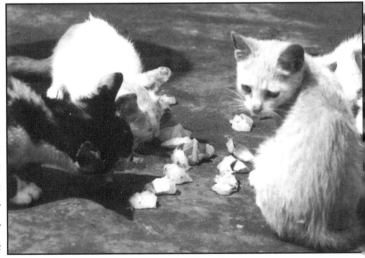

North African kittens enjoy a meal of fresh fish.

our energy and vitality improve.

Protective Chi defends the body against harmful external forces. This Chi is the greatest Yang manifestation in the body. It travels within the chest and abdominal areas, and courses between the skin and muscles. Protective Chi governs the sweat glands and pores, protects skin and hair, and keeps the organs warm. When Protective Chi is abundant, a strong defense system exists, keeping the body safe from harmful outside influences and diseases.

Protective Chi is directly responsible for your cat's immune system. Because of environmental pollution and other forms of external contamination, cats have to have strong Protective Chi to destroy external pathogens and restore balance in the body. Offering your cat Immune System Strengthening acupressure treatments on a regular basis is a good place to start to build your cat's level of natural protection. Acupressure can help cats avoid the "human" diseases that disrupt their natural health.

Meridian Chi is transported through invisible, yet very real, pathways of the meridian system. Chi is constantly carried to the organs and creates an harmonious functioning of all aspects of the human or feline body. It courses through the body every 24 hours.

Current researcher, Robert Becker, M.D., has successfully mapped meridian flows with their acupressure points and determined their specific rhythmic pulses. He has found that pulses consist of 15 minute cycles that overlap a longer twenty-four hour cycle. Additionally, he has discovered that the meridian pathways conduct a current, he hypothesizes that the perineural system acts as a conductor. (Manning, Clark A., *Bioenergetic Medicines East and West*, North Atlantic Books, Berkeley, CA, 1988)

As a touch technique, acupressure works with Meridian Chi to restore the Yin-Yang balance of organ systems, allowing the body to restore and maintain health.

As a touch technique, acupressure works with Meridian Chi to restore the Yin-Yang balance of organ systems, allowing the body to restore and maintain health. By using touch techniques, we remove energy blockages in the meridian pathways so the Chi flows smoothly. We can strengthen, or tonify, a deficient flow of Chi energy through the meridian channels to enhance the movement. When an excessive amount of Chi energy is present, we can sedate, or disperse, the excess Chi as it flows through the meridian pathways.

Chi circulating through the body performs five major functions:
- Generates body warmth.
- Protects the body from external harmful forces.
- Governs the retention of body substances.
- Creates all body movement; it is the source of voluntary and involuntary movement.
- Serves as the basis of organ functions; for example, derives nutrients from food or air, and transforms and transports substances.

When performing an acupressure treatment on your cat, you are manipulating the flow of Chi through the meridian system of his body. Feline Acupressure Treatment, Chapter Three, offers detailed information regarding Meridian Chi and acupressure techniques.

Aspects of Chi

Chi energy, or life force energy, has different aspects. *Shen* represents the spirit aspect of Chi. *Jing* refers to the *life essence* or material aspect of Chi. These fundamental substances are an integral part of Chi and cannot be separated. To the TCM practitioner, Shen and Jing are real, just as a leg and arm are real to a western medical practitioner.

Shen is the creative process that gives rise to thought, emotion, and consciousness. Some people do not believe that cats think and have emotions, but those of us who are "cat people" know they do. Though, a cat's thought process may be simple and primitive, there is much evidence–anecdotal and scientific–that cats think and feel emotions. Any human who has a beloved cat will not hesitate to tell you his or her cat has a full range of emotions from utter joy to heart-stricken grief. Cats definitely are conscious of themselves and the world around them. People who do not know cats often assume we are anthropomorphizing our cats' behaviors. They are simply wrong.

When I play with my cat, who knows whether I do not make her more sport than she makes me?

-Michel De Montaigne

Shen is primarily given to the fetus from both parents, stored in the heart and revealed in the eyes. Shen reflects the interaction of essence and Chi. When the spirit is not balanced, the eyes appear clouded, dull, or vacant. You can tell when your cat is not in full spirit and complete health by looking into his eyes. The harmonious flow of Shen is essential to good health. It needs to be consistently nourished and revitalized.

Consistent acupressure treatments help support and renew a cat's Shen. Acupressure along the Heart Meridian can help replenish the spirit of a depressed or abused animal. Many things contribute to replenishing a cat's Shen, such as rolling in green grass, dancing after a grasshopper, or preening in a sunbeam. Cats need to reconnect with their natural selves regularly to sustain and build Shen.

Combined with Source Chi, Jing or life essence determines the development of each cat's constitution. Jing is regarded as the material, tangible basis of Chi. Jing Chi can be thought of as genetic capability. A kitten's queen and father may be sturdy Maine Coon Cats but if the kitten does not receive quality food and exercise to create Food and Lung Chi, the kitten will not reach full growth potential. Given a healthful, nurturing environment and nourishing food, kittens develop well and attain their genetic potential of Jing.

Jing energy, also called the Source of Life, is stored in the kidneys. It has a fluid nature and circulates throughout the body, along with Chi. Jing determines growth, reproduction, and development. It is involved in producing marrow. In TCM, marrow is broadly defined; it is the substance common to bones, bone marrow, the spinal cord, and the brain. Given this concept of marrow, Jing determines physical and constitutional strength while also impacting concentration and memory.

The fixed quantity of the inherited portions of Source Chi and Jing are the basis of the congenital constitution of the cat. The non-inherited portion of Chi is affected by everyday lifestyle, including exercise, food, and stress level. The best way to positively affect your cat's Jing is to create and environment for a balanced lifestyle. For your cat, this translates to some expression of his predatory instincts, challenging exercise, rest, a natural balanced diet, and healthy living conditions.

Maintaining a balanced flow of Chi, or life force energy, in spirit and physical form is absolutely essential to having a healthy cat. The demands we place on cats to live in our environment causes them stress. A city apartment or a suburban backyard is not a cat's natural habitat. The tamed feline is a tiger in kitty clothing. Consistent acupressure treatments offer cats relief from some of the stress of living in our world, but it would be best to combine them with all of the good things our four-legged friends need.

Yin and Yang

Chi energy, in its many forms and functions, is a dynamic balance between two opposing forces. The concept of Yin and Yang is fundamental to TCM. Theoretically, there is a constant flow between two polarities called Yin and Yang. Within the singular entity of Chi, Yin and Yang are constantly moving and flowing from harmony to disharmony, balance to imbalance. They are opposite of each other and, thus, mutually interdependent; neither can exist without the other. Yin and Yang are constantly in a state of flux, so the increase of one creates the consumption of the other to maintain balance.

The Yin component of Chi is associated with the maintenance and structure of matter while Yang is associated with movement and function. Although the forces of Yin and Yang are not really distinct, they are most clearly differentiated at the extremes. For example, "day" is thought of as Yang, "night" as Yin. In this example, each is clearly defined. As day approaches night, or "dusk", the distinction between Yin and Yang becomes less clear. This is where we see the reality of one dynamic force. Yin and Yang are often represented as opposites. Some of their attributes are:

	YANG	**YIN**
In the world	Excitement	Rest
	Day	Night
	Upper	Lower
	Hollow	Solid
	Sun	Moon
	Positive	Negative
In the body	Spine/back	Chest/Abdomen
	Male	Female
	Protective Chi	Food Chi
	Surface of the body	Interior of the body
	Loud meow	Weak sounds
In disease	Acute	Chronic
	Rapid onset	Gradual onset
	Heat	Cold
	Lies stretched out	Lies curled up
	Constipation	Loose stools
	Thirsty	Not thirsty
	Scanty, dark urination	Profuse, light urination

In a healthy body, Chi circulates through the meridian system channels in an ongoing and self-regulating balance. In an unhealthy body, Chi is not in balance, causing dysfunction. The meridian pathways may be blocked, congested, or stagnated, depending on the indicators or evidence the body is demonstrating. A dysfunction along the meridian pathway reduces your cat's self-regulating, energy-balancing capabilities and can cause a condition of excess or deficient Yin or Yang. Acupressure treatments work to restore the balance of the Chi's Yin/Yang force in your cat's body and to promote healing.

Meridian System - Energy Pathways

Chi energy, in its various forms and functions, provides life and a self-regulating balancing system for a healthy body. The meridians are a network-like channel system that transports Chi to all areas of the body to supply life force energy. The meridian system:

- Moves Chi energy and balances Yin and Yang.
- Reflects signs of disharmony or imbalance.
- Resists external and internal pathogens.
- Regulates conditions of excess and deficiency.

Partial Meridian System Chart

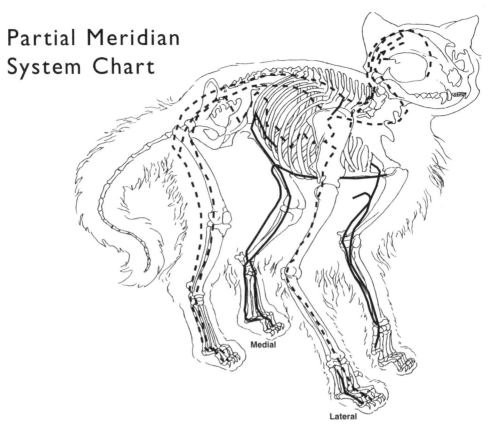

Medial

Lateral

Twelve Major Meridians and Two Extraordinary Vessels

Each of the 12 major meridians is associated with an organ system, transmits Chi, and maintains the balance of the body's systems. The meridians are paired in Yin and Yang couples known as sister meridians. The 12 major organ system meridians are:

YIN	YANG
Lung	Large Intestine
Kidney	Bladder
Liver	Gall Bladder
Heart	Small Intestine
Pericardium	Triple Heater
Spleen	Stomach

There are also eight Extraordinary Vessels or pathways that connect and collect Chi from the 12 major meridians. Unlike the major meridians, these are not linked directly to the 12 organ systems. The Extraordinary Vessels are extremely important because they supplement interactions among the twelve major meridians They also act as reservoirs for the major meridians by absorbing or transferring energy to the twelve major meridians, as needed. For the scope of this book, we discuss only the Extraordinary pathways of the Governing and Conception Vessels, which are the most commonly used and well-known of the Extraordinary Vessels.

The Governing Vessel is known as the *Sea of Yang Channels*. It influences all of the Yang meridians and is used to *tonify* (enhance or strengthen) the body's Yang energy. The Governing Vessel nourishes the brain and spine. Its pathway runs from the anus to the top of the lip on the dorsal, top-side, midline of the cat.

The Conception Vessel is known as the *Sea of Yin Channels*. It influences all of the Yin meridians. The Conception Vessel is very important for the reproductive system of a cat, particularly a queen. It influences her estrous cycle, fertility, pregnancy, and conception. The Conception Vessel's pathway runs from the cat's chin down through the legs, along the mid-line of the chest and belly to just below the anus.

Acupressure and Acupoints

As a revered TCM healing modality, acupressure is similar to acupuncture but does not use needles to stimulate the acupoints along the meridians and other locations. Experience has shown that it is not always necessary to penetrate the surface of the skin to obtain the desired energy-balancing effect. Animals are particularly sensitive and you can perform acupressure sessions between visits to your veterinarian to achieve the maximum healing benefit. Most cats require a fairly light touch and, at times, almost no direct touch.

There are more than 350 acupoints located along the meridians and more than 250 nonmeridian points. Many of these points are located in valleys of the body between muscles and bones. The Chi flows through the meridian channels and is accessible to manipulation through acupressure. When stimulated, the acupressure points along the meridian impacts the flow of Chi energy. During an acupressure treatment, pressure is applied to specific acupoints that either tonifies (increases) or sedates (decreases) Chi energy, as needed, to balance the body and allow healing.

Clark Manning and Louis Vanrenen noted in their book, *Bioenergetic Medicines East and West*:

> Claude Darras, a French medical doctor, has conducted interesting experiments in an attempt to trace the physical effects of acupuncture. When a radioactive isotope is injected into an acupuncture point, it moves away from the point

in a predictable path, following no known anatomical pathways but rather specific acupuncture meridians. Isotopes injected into nonacupuncture point sites do not reproduce this specific motion. Also, when the isotope ceases to move, its movement can be restimulated by needling the point directly beneath the injection.

A comprehensive discussion of the acupoints, their location and purpose, are described in Chapter Five, Feline Acupressure Points. Acupressure treatment techniques for balancing energy through point work are described in Chapter Three, Feline Acupressure Treatment.

Indicators

TCM is a highly refined and flexible system for understanding the body-mind-spirit as a single entity. Although we have transposed the ideas to the feline body, with some reasonable modifications, the basic concepts are the same. TCM strives to determine the underlying cause of an ailment by looking at the entire being from as many perspectives as possible. The practitioner uses his skills of observation to discern fundamental patterns that reveal the root cause of the dysfunctional condition before the course of treatment is developed. TCM practitioners develop their observation skills by learning the Four Examinations of looking, listening and smelling, asking and touching. During the process of gathering information, the practitioner is sorting and classifying the information using three different systems of discerning patterns: Eight Guiding Principles, Six Layers and the Five Phases of Transformation (also known as the Five Element Theory). It takes many years of study and practice to become truly proficient in discerning the patterns of disharmony and arriving at an understanding of the causes of an ailment. For the purposes of this manual, we introduce only the broad concepts behind the theories. The depth and complexity of identifying illnesses and treatments would require a book many times the size of this one.

The Four Examinations

The Four Examinations gives the practitioner a methodology for observing and collecting information about the client. A lot of information can be gathered by looking at a cat and performing a visual inspection. Is his coat dull or shiny? Are his eyes bright or dull? How does he move his body? Does he favor any paw? What does his tongue look like? All of the answers to these questions help the practitioner understand the cat's condition in terms of Yin and Yang.

In Chinese medicine, listening and smelling are connected so they are discussed as a single perspective during an observation phase of understanding the client's ailment. Is the cat's meowing loud and harsh or quiet and soft? Loud vocalization could indicate an excessive and possibly Yang condition. Weak vocalization may indicate a deficient or Yin condition. The TCM practitioner learns the subtleties of smells. Different conditions have characteristic odors. In extreme illness, the odors can become quite pronounced.

The practitioner asks about the client's medical history. In eastern medicine the questioning usually extends beyond what the western doctor would consider reasonable. After learning the basics of the cat's history, the TCM practitioner asks questions having to do with a cat's preference for different times of the year, when is the cat most energetic, what food he likes and dislikes, where the cat selects to sleep. The answers to these questions give the practitioner insights into the cat's basic constitution and attitudes along with medically significant events.

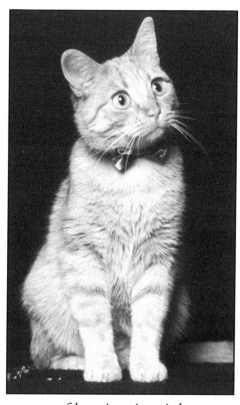

Touch is the fourth area of the examination. The practitioner essentially performs a physical exam by checking energy pulses, meridians, and acupoints then presses areas of the body that may be sensitive, hot or cool, protruding or depressed. This physical examination is highly detailed and complex. Detecting the nature of the energy pulses requires years of learning since it has a language of its own. A teacher characterized the pulses as sort of a computer printout that is available on everyone's wrist. The trick is being able to decode the messages.

During the Four Examinations, the TCM practitioner is collecting a huge amount of data. As this data funnels in, the practitioner carefully processes and categorizes the information. He or she must apply a number of filters through which the information must pass before determining the cause of the imbalance, distinguishing the nature of the pattern of disharmony and, finally, arriving at a comprehensive, holistic course of treatment to pursue.

Eight Guiding Principles

The Eight Guiding Principals, *Ba-gang*, is one of the ways the practitioner sifts and sorts information. It provides further understanding of Yin and Yang. The Eight Guiding Principles are a further extension of Yin and Yang since they are the physical, tangible evidence of Yin and Yang. As the physical representation of polarities of Chi, Yin and Yang provide a method of conceptualizing and distinguishing different patterns.

The practitioner analytically observes the client, using The Four Examinations, to recognize the physical evidence of the Eight Guiding Principles. To identify certain patterns, the practitioner gathers historical, current, and lifestyle information about the cat. Knowing the location, quality, and extent of the eight opposite conditions gives the practitioner a way to clarify and organize the relationship between particular clinical signs.

For example, lethargy and physical weakness in your cat indicate a pattern of Yin deficiency. To make a more precise treatment determination, the TCM practitioner assesses the body's whole condition by observing physical attitude, conformation, areas of swelling, appearance of the skin and coat; and by smelling any unusual odors, and listening to body sounds; noting strength of vocalization. The practitioner then checks particular meridians and acupressure points to see if, to the touch, they are hot or cold, indented or protruding, spongy or dense, painful or benign. Once the practitioner has performed a thorough examination and asked questions about the cat's current condition, lifestyle, and history, he or she discovers the distinguishing pattern, *bian-zheng*, and is able to prepare a treatment plan.

Hard lumps, swelling or dense tissue mass may indicate an excessive Yang condition. Soft lumps, swelling and spongy tissue mass may indicate an excessive Yin condition. In either case, the TCM practitioner continues to observe, collect information, check points, and use other indicators to fully understand the course of treatment required.

Six Layers

The Six Layers is another analytic tool to assist in classifying information gathered during the Four Examinations. There are six energetic layers through which an external influence can pass when Protective Chi and other levels of Chi are not in balance. This causes specific indicators to manifest. For instance, if cold passes into the first layer, your cat may manifest a fever, be afraid of cold or wind, and have a floating pulse. As external pathogens penetrate through the layers, the seriousness of the illness increases. Practitioners in ancient China linked these concepts with The Four Stages, which further expresses the seriousness and life-threatening aspect of the client's illness.

The Five Phases of Transformation

The Five Phases of Transformation, *Wu Xing*, also called the Five Element Theory, brings another level of understanding to the underlying basis of acupressure as a healing art. The Five Phases offer another perspective and explanation of how Chi interacts, balances, and supports all life forms and the world as we know it. This book briefly touches on the intricacies of the Five Phases, since they are one of the most significant conceptual foundations of TCM. Many other books are devoted to narrow slices of the subject because The Five Phases of Transformation is such a large body of knowledge.

Metaphorically, the Five Phases are identified as Metal, Water, Wood, Fire and Earth. Sometimes referred to as elements, these Phases are primal forms that are the basis of all that exists in life. Each Phase, or element, is part of a larger, ordered transformational phase or cycle of existence in which nothing is static. The Creation Cycle, moving clockwise around the circle, is the building or growth cycle and represents a continuous flow of nourishing energy. Unending growth would cause an exponential compounding of energy from one phase to another, resulting in a dangerously extreme imbalance. The Control Cycle counteracts the Creation Cycle, constantly interacting to restore balance and harmonious synchronicity among all things.

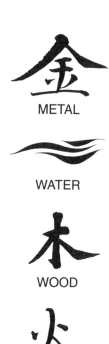

METAL

WATER

WOOD

FIRE

EARTH

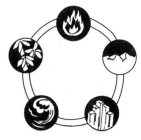

Traditional description of the Creation Cycle:

Fire creates Earth	Ashes of fire add to earth.
Earth creates Metal	Adding earth creates metal.
Metal creates Water	Metal separates, allowing water to flow.
Water creates Wood	Water nourishes the growth of wood.
Wood creates Fire	Wood fuels fire.

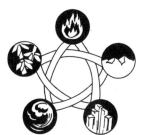

Traditional description of the Controlling Cycle:

Fire controls Metal	Heat of fire melts metal.
Metal controls Wood	Metal chops wood.
Wood controls Earth	Roots of trees grow through earth.
Earth controls Water	Earth dams water.
Water controls Fire	Water dowses fire.

Creation & Controlling Cycle

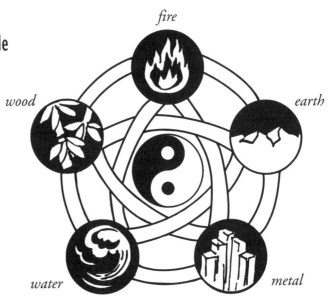

The Five Phases of Transformation is a conceptual framework that describes and defines the changes and relationships in all of nature, including animals. The Phases are associated with the seasons, stages of transformative existence, climate, Yin and Yang organ systems, body tissue, geographic direction, predominant emotion, taste, smell, sense organ, color–everything!

FIVE PHASES OF TRANSFORMATIONAL CORRESPONDENCE CHART

	METAL	WATER	WOOD	FIRE	EARTH
TRANSITION	Harvest	Storage	Birth	Growth/Creation	Maturity
SEASON	Fall	Winter	Spring	Summer	Late Summer
CLIMATE	Dry/Wind	Cold	Windy	Hot	Wet/Humid
DIRECTION	West	North	East	South	Center
COLOR	White	Blue	Green	Red	Yellow
EMOTION	Grief	Fear	Anger	Joy	Sympathy/Worry
SENSORY ORIFICE	Nose	Genitals/Ears	Eyes	Tongue	Mouth
SMELL	Putrid	Rotten	Rank	Burning	Fragrant/Sweet
GOVERNED PART OF BODY	Skin & Body Hair	Bones & Marrow	Tendons & Ligaments	Vascular System	Muscles & Lymph
MERIDIANS	Lung & Large Intestine	Kidney & Bladder	Liver & Gall Bladder	Heart & Small Intestine Pericardium & Triple Heater	Spleen & Stomach

The Five Phases provide essential information for the acupressure practitioner by directing the selection of appropriate meridians and specific points needed to rebalance and restore harmony between the internal and external worlds. Each set of meridians is associated with one of the Five Phases. The elements and their corresponding Yin/Yang meridians are:

ELEMENT	MERIDIAN	
	Yin	**Yang**
Metal	Lung	Large Intestine
Water	Kidney	Bladder
Wood	Liver	Gall Bladder
Fire	Heart	Small Intestine
	Pericardium	Triple Heater
Earth	Spleen	Stomach

Human and feline bodies are microcosms. We are composed of the same elements as the rest of the world. The Five Phases are always present in our bodies, by way of our organs and the meridians they impact. If Chi energy is blocked or imbalanced while traveling through the body, dysfunction and disease can manifest. Using the conceptual base of the Eight Guiding Principles and Five Phases, a practitioner can identify: (1) where the blockage has occurred (2) if the energy is deficient or excessive (3) which meridians and acupoints need to be manipulated. As a result of the acupressure treatment, the blockage is resolved and the energy can flow freely, allowing the body to heal.

For example, skin problems in your cat could indicate a deficiency in the Lung and/or Large Intestine Meridians (see Correspondence Chart for Governed Part of the Body). To identify points for tonifying or strengthening these meridians, the practitioner looks at the Creation Cycle–Earth creates, or strengthens, Metal. When the Earth Points on the Lung and Large Intestine Meridians–Lu 9 and LI 11–are stimulated they strengthen skin.

If a queen is cycling excessively, look at the Kidney Meridian to sedate the cycling activity (see Correspondence Chart for Orifices). The estrous cycle is partially a function governed by the Kidney Meridian, which is a water element. To "control" this, look at the Control Cycle–Earth controls Water. The practitioner then considers sedating the Earth points in the Kidney and Bladder meridians, Ki 3 and Bl 54, to disperse the excess energy. (Note: Lu 9, LI 11, Ki 3, and Bl 54 are examples of Command Points. Classification of points is discussed further in Chapter Five, Feline Acupressure Points.

Five Phases and Qualities

The Five Phases represent distinct physical qualities and characteristics; they also point to attributes of personality and temperament. Think of cats as an expression of a certain element. Any breed or natural-selection cat can be identified as having predominant physical constitutions and temperaments.

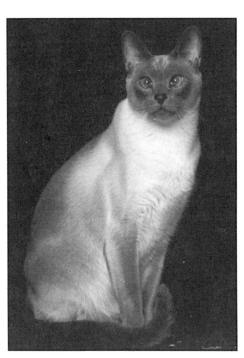

Metal Cat

Cats with balanced "metal" constitutions appear to have a healthy, slow, fluidity in their body movements. They particularly enjoy the temperature and quality of light in the autumn. There are times when Metal Cats seem to be sorrowfully grieving a lost friend. They often have respiratory and immune system issues. These cats are soft, loving, quiet, and serious.

Water Cat

Balanced Water Cats have beautiful, shiny, healthy coats with strong, dense, large-boned bodies. They tend to have a lot of physical energy. Even with all their physical prowess, these cats can appear to be hyper-vigilant, extremely observant, and even timid at times. In the wild, this feline is seen as a survivor, self-sufficient, and resilient. A Water Cat has keen senses and is able-bodied but must work at not having fear overwhelm him.

Wood Cat

Wood Cats are usually angular and lean, energetic, strong and free-moving. They can be seen as independent and aloof around humans. Around other cats they are somewhat aggressive and very expressive. They tend to be more active in the spring and take full advantage of the season to prove their excellent hunting skills.

Fire Cat

In TCM terms, a Fire Cat with a balanced "fire" constitution exhibits a joyful and vibrant personality. He is charismatic, playful, and friendly. The Fire Cat moves with the grace of an athlete and demonstrates an eagerness to try new challenges, he is a natural hunter. His warm, gentle nature endears him to people.

Earth Cat

Cats with a balanced "earth" constitution tend to have broad, strong bodies. They are loyal, emotionally empathetic, and, at times, seem worried. The Earth Cat is usually a good eater and runs the risk of being overweight. These cats land heavily on all four paws when they jump off the furniture. The Earth Cat has a steady, tolerant nature and exhibits a calm and grounded demeanor. These cats like small children and make good family cats.

Though your cat could care less about Traditional Chinese Medicine's conceptual base, we wanted to give you some exposure to it because it offers a fascinating and unending exploration in natural healing. *Acu-Cat* is intended to make acupressure accessible to people who want to communicate their caring intention to their cats.

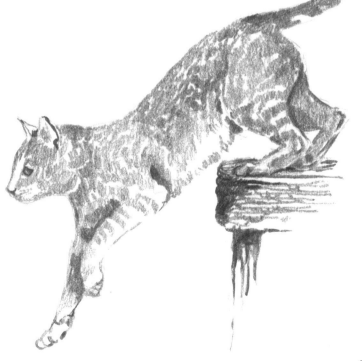

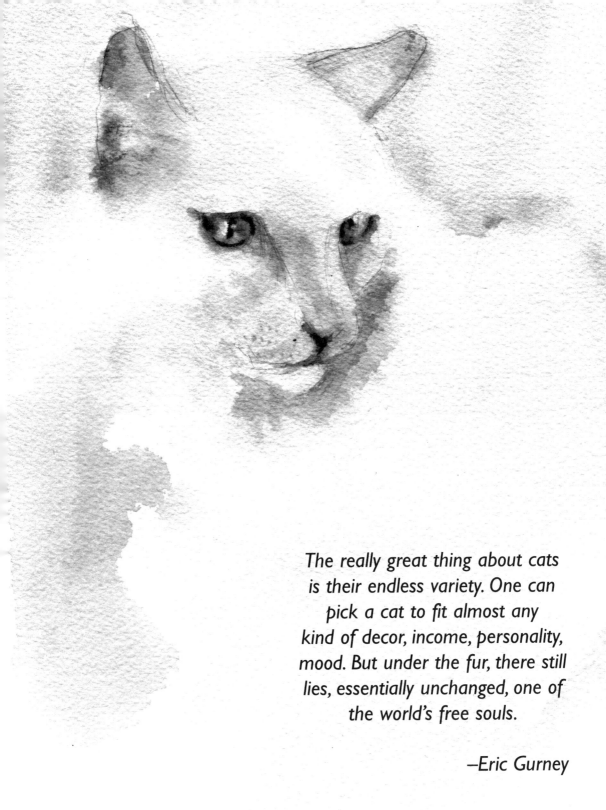

The really great thing about cats
is their endless variety. One can
pick a cat to fit almost any
kind of decor, income, personality,
mood. But under the fur, there still
lies, essentially unchanged, one of
the world's free souls.

—Eric Gurney

chapter three
Feline Acupressure Treatment

Let all of life's pressures wash away. Touch your cat's soft shoulder, feel his warmth and responsiveness. Take three deep breaths, look out the window, then pick up a toy and catch your cat's attention. A few minutes of enjoying and playing prepares you both for an acupressure treatment.

The acupressure treatment starts when you and your cat connect. These moments can take many shapes and forms. When your cat is relaxed and purring on the couch next to you, or when your bouncy kitten has played "ferocious tiger" for the past hour and is ready for a nap–these are good times to begin a session.

An acupressure treatment is a dynamic, energetic interaction between two equal partners–you and your cat. Your role is to hold a clear intention of enhancing his well-being. To accomplish this, you must be consciously present and use your knowledge, experience, and intuition throughout the treatment process. The other half of the partnership is your cat's innate ability to feel energetic sensations in his body and his capacity to communicate with you through body language.

It may take a few sessions of just becoming relaxed and comfortable with each other since intentional touch is different from simple petting and affection. Additionally, cats do not like to be restrained in any way and it would be counter productive to have a frantic cat scrambling to get away. Once your cat becomes accustomed to having acupressure treatments, he will regard it as a treat! Your cat is very aware of when you are attuned to his needs. In turn, he will help guide you through a treatment–if you are alert to the directions he gives you. Allowing your cat to communicate what he needs is a significant part of sharing an acupressure treatment.

A complete acupressure treatment session is divided into three parts: before, during, and after. The key to performing a successful acupressure treatment is to pay attention to your cat, with healing intent, while working through each segment of the treatment.

Acupressure Treatment

Pre-Treatment (Before)
      Selecting a location
      When not to perform an acupressure treatment
      Preparing yourself
      Introducing yourself and gaining permission to treat
      Observing your cat before treatment
Phases of the Acupressure Treatment (During)
      Observing your cat during treatment
      Phases of an acupressure treatment:
         Opening
         Point work
         Closing
Post Treatment (After)

Pre-Treatment

Selecting a Treatment Location

To achieve the best results, select a place where your cat feels safe and relaxed. Most cats are comfortable in their own living area. If your cat has a special bed, rug or sunny spot, it is fine to work with him there. Let him choose whether he wants to lie down, sit or stand. Allow him to decide which direction to face during the treatment. You do not want to restrict your cat's ability to move around during the treatment because he will be giving you cues about how he is feeling, plus, most cats dislike being restricted.

Pick a time of day when your cat has had enough exercise and isn't hungry. The quieter and calmer the environment, the better.

Make sure you are comfortable, too. You might have to shift your position fairly often during the treatment; it helps pre-

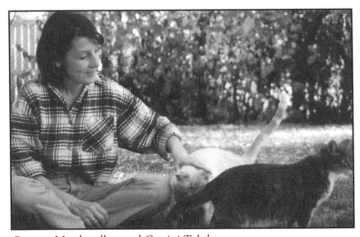

Donna, Marshmallow and Gemini Tukel

vent stress on your muscles and joints. An acupressure treatment needs to be pleasurable for both of you. Consider the possibility of your cat reacting to some of the points that may be tender to the touch. For your own safety, if you know your cat has a tendency to scratch or bite, be careful. If your cat has you in his grip, just relax your hand, play dead and he will most likely release you. This feline reaction harkens back to a cat's instinct to kill living prey.

Other pets in the household usually enjoy being in the same environment where energetic work is being done. They receive benefit from a treatment by just being in the room. Most often, the other cats and dogs will lie near where you are working and go to sleep, sending calming signals to the cat receiving the treatment.

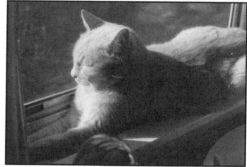

Fozzie Peterson

When Not to Perform an Acupressure Treatment

There are times when acupressure treatments are contraindicated. The purpose of an acupressure treatment is to rebalance the body's Chi energy. But there are specific times when the body needs to focus energy in a particular way, and interfering with the energy flow could be harmful. During pregnancy, the body's energy is naturally out of balance and needs to stay that way for the duration of the pregnancy. When you have a pregnant queen, acupressure treatments are not recommended. In Chapter Six, Acupressure Treatments for Specific Conditions, particular acupressure points that are not to be used during pregnancy are identified.

Do not perform an acupressure treatment:
• Just after feeding; wait three to four hours before beginning a treatment.
• After a lot of exercise; wait until your cat is calm.
• When your cat has a high fever; call your veterinarian immediately.
• If your cat has an infectious disease; call your veterinarian immediately.
• After a male has expelled semen; wait twelve hours before a treatment.
• When your queen is pregnant; resume treatments after delivery.

Preparing Yourself

To achieve the highest quality treatment, you need to feel connected to your own Chi energy and become centered within yourself before beginning. Clearing your mind of the day's demands and activities will help you focus your energy and create your healing intent. To clear your mind of distracting thoughts, do the following breathing exercise:

- Sit quietly for several moments and picture your thoughts as clouds floating out of view.
- Breathe in Chi energy from the air and feel it moving through your lungs and down into your abdomen.
- Hold the Chi in your abdomen for several seconds and feel its balancing properties.
- Exhale and follow the vibration of your breath as it moves across the room.
- Repeat this exercise for eight breaths.

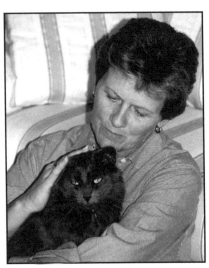

Jan introduces herself and gains permission to work on Fredd.

After completing the breathing exercise, slowly focus and feel your own energy. Then picture your cat and conceptualize your intent to assist in his healing process. These simple activities will increase your awareness of your own Chi energy, reduce tension in your body, and heighten your ability to feel your cat's energy.

Introducing Yourself and Gaining Permission

Cats appreciate it if you say hello before you begin an acupressure treatment. Take a moment to talk to your cat while gently touching and stroking him. When you feel connected, ask him, either aloud or to yourself, if you can give him a treatment, then wait for a response. Signs of his acceptance are: turning toward you, softening his eyes, moving his body into yours, or communicating energetically. If you receive no response, ask again. If he does not respond on the second request, move with him to a different location and ask again. If you still receive no response, honor you cat's choice. Having a cat give no response usually means he simply does not want body work at this time. Ask again on another day.

Observing Your Cat

Observation is an art. It requires all of your attention and perception. Use all of your senses, intuition, and knowledge of your cat. When observing your cat with this level of intensity, you will be able to develop a baseline of information for treatment. Additionally, you will have information for comparison with subsequent treatments. We suggest that you keep a record of your treatments, noting any changes.

Observations

Look at your cat's body objectively and ask yourself the following questions:

What is his general demeanor?

Are his eyes dull or bright?

Is he over or under weight?

What is the condition of his coat?

Is his coat dull, lifeless, dry, or shiny?

Are there any bare spots on his coat?

Are there areas he has been scratching?

What is the condition of his claws?

Are there any unusual odors?

Is he alert and listening to you?

Does he appear to be in pain?

Are there any signs of recent injury?

Ask the following questions while watching your cat in motion:

Are his movements smooth?

Is his reach even on both the right and left sides of his body?

Does he show any stiffness in his joints?

Does he favor one leg or one side?

Does he hold his head erect and straight?

Acupressure Treatment

Observing Your Cat During Treatment

Your cat may respond to acupressure in obvious and subtle ways. Obvious reactions could be muscle spasms, licking, salivating, panting, chewing, or yawning more than usual. Other reactions include moving away from or into the point of pressure, stretching, seeing a distinct change in his breathing pattern, or hearing a change in the loudness of purring, or scratching or licking himself on a particular area of his body. Record his energetic reactions because they are clues to understanding the rebalancing of energy your cat is experiencing.

Equally important are the more subtle signs your cat may display during a treatment. Note changes in his facial expressions, such as softening of the eyes or relaxing of the mouth, chin, or ears. Notice any abdominal sounds. Many of these are signs of energy release along a meridian.

As you sharpen your skills of observation, the list of your cat's reactions will expand. Your awareness of the cat's body and its healing process will grow as you pay close attention to all of the changes.

Maintaining a record of your cat's reactions to an acupressure treatment is an important tool for developing your skills of observation. By recording reactions, you have information for future treatments and benchmarks for understanding past behaviors and health conditions. Having a record is useful when discussing your cat's health with your veterinarian. A detailed outline for a Treatment Log is included in Chapter Seven, Maintenance Treatment.

Acupressure Treatment Phases

Within the treatment segment of the entire acupressure treatment are three phases:

- Opening
- Point Work
- Closing

A complete acupressure session usually includes stretch exercises as a fourth phase. Cats, by both their nature and size, are not good candidates for human-assisted stretch exercises. They love to stretch with gloriously languid movements without help. Most cats tend to resist our helping them extend and contract their limbs. Because of their size and temperament, we recommend excluding stretching in an acupressure treatment for cats.

As you progress through each of these treatment phases, relax and be receptive to the energetic messages your cat is giving you. Remember to clear your mind and center your energy so you can concentrate on your healing intent. Allow your breathing to become deep and relaxed; this will assist in balancing your cat's Chi and help promote the healing effect.

Set aside enough time for the treatment so you will not feel rushed. As you gain competence, you will be able to complete a treatment in less time. Generally, the duration of a complete treatment is 20 to 30 minutes: for the Opening phase, allow approximately 5 minutes; for Point Work, 10-20 minutes and for the Closing, 5 minutes.

Opening

The Opening prepares your cat for bodywork. It enhances his awareness of his body and allows him to relax and become comfortable with structured, intentional touch.

To Open using the smooth hand technique or the index/middle finger technique, gently position the heel of your hand or index and middle fingers in full contact with your cat's body. Apply about one-quarter to one-half of a pound of pressure with the heel of your hand, relaxing your fingers. Start on the upper part of your cat's neck. Stroke down along the Bladder Meridian (see next page) from the neck to the shoulders. Depending on your cat's size, the Bladder Meridian runs about one-half to one finger width off the spine on either side of his body.

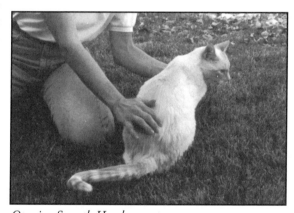

Opening Smooth Hand

Continue to apply pressure and stroke over the back, gliding along the rump, down the gluteal muscles and hamstrings. Follow the contour of the back of the leg to the hock and stay lateral from there all the way down to the paw. Repeat this Opening procedure two or three times on both sides of the cat's body. The slow but fluid pace at which you Open expresses your intent in a calming manner.

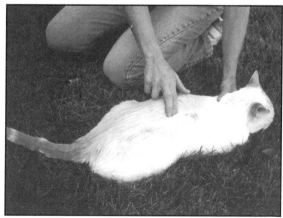

Index and Middle Finger Opening

39

Bladder
Meridian

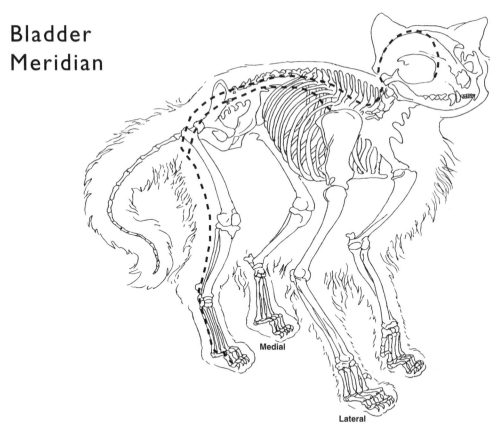

Medial

Lateral

While performing the Opening, distinguish the differences in your cat's body temperature and muscle tone. Notice surface protrusions and depressions. When there is a deficiency, acupressure points along the meridian often feel like soft, spongy depressions. When the Chi energy is excessive, points can feel rigid and resistant to the touch. These findings will help guide you when doing the acupoint work discussed in the next section. Record reactions and observations in your Treatment Log for the Opening phase of the treatment.

Point Work Concepts

Point Work is the second phase of an acupressure treatment and its foundation. The intent of Point Work is to stimulate specific acupoints along a meridian, to balance the cat's energy and promote an environment for healing. By stimulating specific, individual acupoints along a meridian, you release energy blocks. If the Chi energy is excessive, you need to sedate or disperse the energy so the natural flow of Chi resumes. If the Chi is deficient along the meridian, you need to draw more energy to it by tonifying and strengthening the acupressure point to resolve the deficiency. When energy is harmoniously balanced, the body's natural ability to heal is restored.

Acupressure points, also called *acupoints*, have specific qualities and characteristics. They most often are located in valleys of the body, in depressions next to or between muscles and bones, and in the areas surrounding joints. See Chapter Five, Feline Acupressure Points, for further information regarding the function and attributes of acupoints.

Selecting the Point Work for an acupressure treatment begins during the Opening segment of a treatment. While performing the Opening, focus on finding areas of energy blocks and observe reactions your cat may have to your touch. A spontaneous pain reaction at any point may indicate an imbalance in that meridian. Tenderness revealed by light pressure indicates excessive Chi energy. Tenderness revealed by slightly heavier pressure or a soft, cool feeling to a point may indicate an area deficient in Chi energy.

When energy is harmoniously balanced, the body's natural ability to heal is restored.

Learning the characteristics of acupoints is extremely important. The amount of knowledge needed to have a comprehensive grasp of the concepts related to acupoints and acupressure treatments is beyond the scope of this manual. Many people not fully versed in the depth and complexity of Traditional Chinese Medicine have applied acupressure treatments and received positive results. The following description of acupoints offers you a way to discern some of their attributes. We suggest you review the bibliography included in this book to help continue your study and gain a greater understanding of Traditional Chinese Medicine.

The feel, texture, and temperature of an acupoint provides information about that point. Points are considered either "excess" or "deficient." As your proficiency in feeling energy improves, you will become increasingly aware of the distinctions between the two. Points may exhibit the following attributes:

EXCESS ACUPOINTS	DEFICIENT ACUPOINTS
Protruding	Depressed
Warm	Cool or Cold
Painful or Sensitive	Vacant or Empty
Tender to light pressure	Tender to deep pressure
Hard or Dense	Soft or Spongy
Acute	Chronic

Point Work

When an acupoint has an excess of Chi, it may protrude and feel warm to the touch. Often, it is sensitive to light pressure. Your cat may react by showing signs of discomfort when you touch that point. Excessive points need to be sedated and the energy dispersed. To sedate a point, apply light pressure, feel for a line or place of resistance and stop applying pressure at that level until the resistance dissolves. Then apply slightly more pressure until you again feel some resistance. Wait until the resistance dissolves and exert a little more pressure. The process of sedating a point may take as long as five minutes, so be patient and proceed slowly.

If the excess point is very tender, work the points located in front of it and behind it on the same meridian. This will help balance the energy of the meridian and release some of the blocked energy of that point. Once the adjacent points have been sedated, your cat may allow you to work the original excess point.

When a point is deficient in energy, it will often palpate as a depression, be cool or cold, and feel soft to the touch. The point may be tender to deep pressure. A deficient point usually indicates a chronic condition as opposed to an acute condition. When a point feels deficient, strengthen or tonify the energy. To tonify a point, apply pressure in short, pulsating thumb movements. Tonifying a point takes less time than sedating a point. A good indication of sufficient stimulation to a deficient point is a warming of that point.

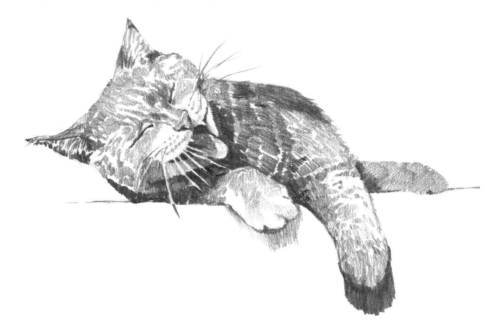

Muddy Water
....Another way of understanding acupressure point work

Plunge your hand into a smooth-water pond and quickly reach for the silt-layered bottom.
Spirals of small particles lift up filling the undercurrents of water.
The disturbed water muddies and you lose sight of your hand.
What was on the bottom is lost to your sight and touch.

Gently cut the surface of the motionless pond.
Slowly, evenly, glide down to the bottom.
Lightly touch the first silt layer with the tip of your thumb.
Feel the temperature of the place your thumb tip is resting.
Sense the energy in that place.
Is it a dull, depressed, empty, cool point?
Is it hot, protruding, angry?
Is it calm, mild, simply smooth to the touch?

The dull, cool, vacant place needs warming attention.
Bring energy to that point.
Lightly move your thumb in a clockwise circular direction and move on.

Angry, hot points request sensitive care.
Not disturbing the surrounding water, add a bit of pressure.
The tip of your thumb moves one layer down into the silt.
What do you feel?
Resistance?
Do not press on. Stop, let up ever so slightly.
Stay the course, hold the point with intention.
Wait for the resistant barrier of energy to pass on, it will.
Move back into the point, is the resistance gone?
Are there more layers of resistance?
Is it more like a multi-layered onion than a silt-bottomed pond?

No reason to rush; energy moves at its own pace.
Each level of resistance takes its time merging back into the harmonious flow of all that exists.
Every toneless point fills and flows into the universal river of life force energy.
Your touch and loving intention are gifts to all that is, was, and will ever be.

43

Point Work Techniques

There are three Point Work techniques recommended for feline acupressure:

- Direct thumb pressure technique
- Pulsing thumb technique
- Circular thumb technique

Experiment with each of the three Point Work techniques. Practice them on a willing friend to become more proficient before working on your cat. The thumb is most commonly selected for Point Work because it is neutral in polarity, that is, it does not have a positive or negative force field. In places where it is awkward to use your thumb, place your middle finger on top of your index finger to achieve neutral polarity. By applying neutral polarity to acupoints, you can avoid the possibility of further accentuating an imbalance by the addition of a positive or negative charge.

Be sure to modify your technique in relation to the size of your cat.

Synchronize your breathing pattern with the stimulation of points. Breathe out while easing into the point, breathe in while slowly releasing the point. After a few treatments, your cat is likely to synchronize his breathing with yours.

Move into a point with very light body pressure. This ensures a smoothness of motion. Be sure to modify this technique based on the size of your cat. Kittens or small, delicate-boned cats require only ounces of pressure. Larger cats will accept up to half a pound of pressure. Initially, apply light pressure then slowly increase the amount of pressure as your cat permits.

After a few weeks of regular acupressure treatments, most cats begin to tell you which points need work. Watch your cat's body language; he will tell you the points needing work by touching a point with his nose, by moving his body into a point you are working, or by scratching or licking a particular point. Cats are highly attuned to body work and quickly understand we are contributing to their health and well-being. This is a wonderful form of communication and connection you can have with your cat.

General Guidelines For Acupoint Work

- Point Work is performed generally from front to rear and top to bottom.
- Keep both hands on your cat while giving a treatment. One hand does the Point Work while the other feels reactions such as muscle spasms or twitches and releases. The hand not doing Point Work also serves to soothe your cat and acts as an energy connection.
- Breathe out while moving into a point; breathe in when letting up on the point.
- Apply pressure gently as you ease into a point and slowly release out of a point. All movements must be smooth and even -- no abrupt changes in pressure. Start by applying light pressure, taking your cat's size into consideration, and increasing the pressure only as your cat allows.
- Apply pressure at a 90-degree angle to the meridian line on which you are working.

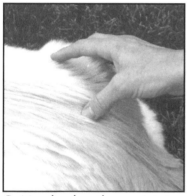

Position thumb on the acupoint at a 90° angle to the meridian. Gently put direct pressure into the point.

Direct Thumb Pressure

To perform Point Work using the direct thumb technique, place the ball of your thumb on the acupressure point perpendicular to its meridian. Gently apply direct pressure (approximately one-quarter to one-half pound of pressure; modify pressure in relation to the size of the cat) to the point while breathing out. Slowly release the point while breathing in and move to the next point.

Pulsing Thumb Technique

A firm, slow pulsing thumb motion sedates or disperses excessive Chi energy. A light, fast pulsing motion tonifies or strengthens a deficient area by drawing energy into the point and surrounding area. While using the pulsating thumb technique, strive to maintain rhythmic movements.

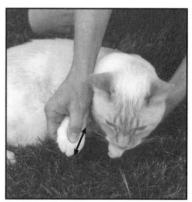

Position thumb same as Direct Thumb Technique. Pulsate lightly to tonify. A heavier pulsing motion sedates.

Circular Thumb Technique

Begin with the direct thumb pressure technique. After easing into the point, continue to apply pressure while rotating your thumb in a circular motion. Clockwise rotation tonifies or strengthens energy. Counterclockwise motion sedates or disperses energy. Complete 3–6 full revolutions before moving to the next point.

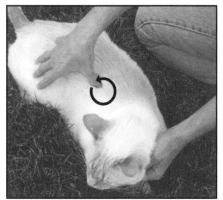

Clockwise Circular Thumb to tonify point.

Counter-Clockwise Circular Thumb to sedate a point.

Closing

The Closing, phase three of the acupressure treatment, has two purposes: (1) it reinforces the energy flow between the points on the same meridians stimulated during point work; and (2) it establishes a healthy cellular memory pattern.

During the Closing we are reinforcing the energy along the entire meridian system and helping to maintain the state achieved during Point Work. Cellular memory is the cell's learned response to a chronic stimulus such as pain. Over the 24 four hour period following an acupressure treatment, the cell's previously learned negative responses are replaced with a positive response.

Smooth Hand or
Index/Middle Finger Closings

For feline acupressure treatments, we suggest using either a smooth hand closing or index/middle finger techniques. Experiment with the two techniques and select the one, or combination of techniques, that is best for you and your cat.

To perform a Closing using the smooth hand technique, position the heel of your hand in contact with your cat. For the index/middle finger closing, place your middle finger on top of your index finger. With either technique,

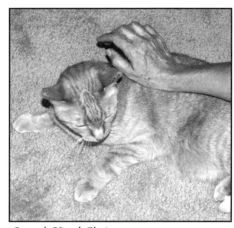

Smooth Hand Closing

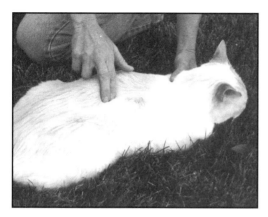

Index/Middle Finger Closing

exert light pressure and glide your hand over your cat's body from front to rear and top to bottom.

Begin at the neck, go over the shoulders, across the back, and over the hind quarters. Continue down the back leg, past the hock, completing the Closing at the end of the cat's paw.

Post-Treatment

After a complete acupressure treatment, the Chi energy flow in your cat's body is changing, his body awareness has shifted, and blockages in his meridian pathways have been released. Your cat is experiencing new and different physical sensations. He may be calm and want to rest for a while. Completion of the rebalancing of energy takes about 24 hours after an acupressure treatment.

General Guidelines For Closing
- Closing work is performed from front to rear and top to bottom.
- Keep both hands on your cat while Closing. One hand does the Closing work, the other serves to calm your cat and acts as a connection.
- Movements are smooth and without any abrupt changes in pressure.
- Complete the Closing technique twice for all of the meridians worked during the treatment on both sides of your cat's body.

General Post-Treatment Guidelines
- After a treatment, your cat may appear "worse" before he feels better. Chi energy flows through the body on a 24-hour cycle and it can take a complete cycle to experience the benefits of the treatment.
- Check your cat every two-to-three hours and record in your Treatment Log any changes in behavior, movement, or mannerisms.

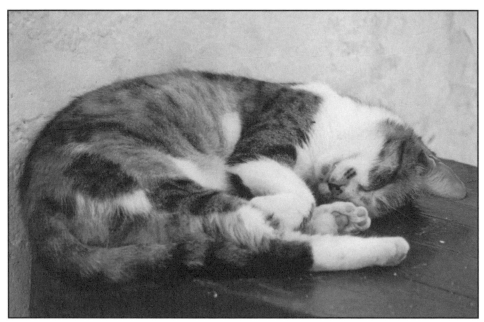

Photo: Elisabeth Apt, Haifa, Israel

Cats are rather delicate creatures and they are subject to a good many ailments, but I never heard of one who suffered from insomnia.
— Joseph Wood Krutch

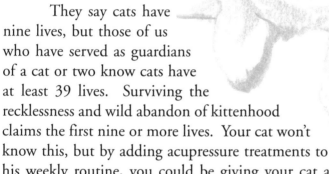

chapter four
Feline Meridian System

They say cats have nine lives, but those of us who have served as guardians of a cat or two know cats have at least 39 lives. Surviving the recklessness and wild abandon of kittenhood claims the first nine or more lives. Your cat won't know this, but by adding acupressure treatments to his weekly routine, you could be giving your cat a chance at a few more lives. Don't tell him or he might go out and jump off a roof top just to see if it works.

Meridians

Chi flows through the human and feline bodies along pathways or channels called meridians. They can be viewed as three-dimensional force fields that travel throughout the body. Chi moves through the meridians, transporting nourishment, strength, and healing properties. The meridian system connects and unifies the entire body, linking internal organs and external body. In Chinese medicine, we constantly strive to maintain a naturally balanced state within the meridian system. When the meridians are balanced and the Chi is flowing smoothly, health and self-healing takes place.

I love cats because I enjoy my home, and little by little, they become its visible soul.
– Jean Cocteau

49

Since the Chi circulates through the meridian system and connects the interior with the exterior of the cat's body, we can influence the flow of Chi by touching various points–known as acupressure points or acupoints–along a meridian.

In both humans and cats, the meridian system consists of twelve major bilateral meridians. Each of these meridians is associated with a specific organ system. In addition to the twelve major meridians, there are eight, non-paired, Extraordinary Vessels. The eight Extraordinary Vessels do not have an organ sys-

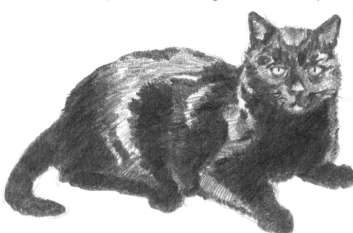

tem directly associated with them. Two of these–the Governing Vessel and the Conception Vessel–are considered part of the major meridian system partially because they have acupressure points that are not on any other meridian.

Meridian Imbalance

When the Chi energy flowing through a meridian is not in balance the entire meridian system does not flow harmoniously. This lack of harmony affects the entire body and its relationship to its natural environment.

Meridian theory is based on the belief that when there is a blockage or some form of interruption along a meridian pathway where the Chi does not flow smoothly, it will cause an imbalance or disharmony. An imbalance can cause a local dysfunction and eventually a disease in the organ associated with the meridian. For example, a disharmony in the Triple Heater Meridian may manifest as a shoulder ache because the Triple Heater Meridian passes through the shoulder. A disharmony in the Gall Bladder Meridian may appear as a sciatic problem since the Gall Bladder Meridian travels through the hip and down the back leg. If imbalances are left untreated, physical discomfort becomes more severe and tissue changes can manifest.

In TCM, an imbalance in a meridian is either a condition of excess or deficient Chi. Blocked, congested, or stagnated Chi is caused by external and internal influences. An external influence would be a cold, damp wind while an internal influence may be extreme anger. Once a disharmony in the meridian system occurs, the TCM practitioner uses many indicators to assess the animal's condition and understand the cause of the disharmony before arriving at a course of treatment.

Meridian Organ Systems

From an energetic point of view, an organ is not merely the organ itself. The entire organ system is responsible for the impact or sphere of influence the organ has on the entire body. For instance, while the Heart Meridian governs the entire vascular system, it also is the center of emotional and mental consciousness and other brain functions. Since the Heart Meridian rules mental energy, it is responsible for Shen, the spirit Chi of the animal.

Each organ system governs a particular part of the body, soft tissues, emotions, and functions. Other names for the organ systems are Zang-Fu Organs. The Zang Organs are Yin Organs that tend to be dense and are responsible for storing and transforming body substances. The Fu Organs are Yang and tend to be hollow and transport nutrients and body waste. The Zang-Fu Organs function to maintain the harmonious flow of Chi energy through the meridians.

ZANG / YIN	FU / YANG
Lung	Large Intestine
Kidney	Bladder
Liver	Gall Bladder
Heart	Small Intestine
Pericardium	Triple Warmer
Spleen	Stomach

Zang-Fu Organs are paired as sister meridians. One of the pair is a Yin, the other is a Yang. The Zang/Yin sister meridians flow along the underside, or ventral aspect, of the cat's body while the Fu/Yang sister meridians travel along the top, or dorsal aspect, of the cat's body. Lung and Large Intestine are sister meridians. The Lung Meridian is the Zang/Yin meridian and the Large Intestine is the Fu/Yang meridian. Often, sister meridians are worked on during the same acupressure treatment, because one is the reflection of the other. If one sister meridian has an excess of Chi, the other will have a deficiency of Chi. Working with one or both of the sister meridians can resolve an imbalance.

Chi Energy along the Meridians

Chi circulates through the meridian system once every 24 hours. Chi energy is concentrated for approximately two hours in each of the twelve major meridians. During these periods of energy concentration, stimulating the acupressure points along the meridian associated with the time period will produce more powerful results. For instance, if there is a condition that indicates a Small Intestine imbalance, working acupressure points along the Small Intestine Meridian will have a stronger effect between one and three in the afternoon.

No "Right" Location

The exact locations of feline and human meridians vary, depending on the source. It is difficult to identify a "right" location. Meridian drawings are a guide, not an exact road map.

Learning to feel the energy along the meridians will help develop your "energy awareness." Begin by tracing the meridian lines on your cat, using the charts as a guide. Trace each meridian several times until you feel the energy-flow pattern, while your cat enjoys this new sensory experience.

We usually recommend working the Liver Meridian points if your cat seems to be consistently angry and agitated (an excess wood condition). However, awakening at one or two in the morning to enhance the therapeutic nature of the Liver flow might cause you to be agitated and out of sorts, so we suggest you find a more convenient time to perform an acupressure session.

Learning the Meridians

We suggest you become familiar with all the meridians. The best way to learn the location of each of the twelve meridians and the two Extraordinary Vessels is to take a half an hour daily for a week to trace them on your cat. Find a location where you and your cat are comfortable and safe–a soft grassy area, carpeted floor, or comfortable arm chair. Make sure you do not strain any part of your body while working with your cat. Place the heel of your hand or your index and middle finger down on the cat. Lightly stroke your cat, tracing the line of each meridian. The more familiar you are with the meridian pathways, the more readily you will understand and perform an acupressure treatment. This also is a good way to prepare your cat for the new sensory experiences of an acupressure treatment.

Direction and Time Flow of Chi Energy Along Meridians

Zang/Yin Meridians	Fu/Yang Meridians
Lung Meridian 3 - 5 AM	Large Intestine Meridian 5 - 7 AM
Spleen Meridian 9 - 11 AM	Stomach Meridian 7 - 9 AM
Heart Meridian 11 - 1 PM	Small Intestine Meridian 1 - 3 PM
Kidney Meridian 5 - 7 PM	Bladder Meridian 3 - 5 PM
Pericardium Meridian 7 - 9 PM	Triple Heater Meridian 9 - 11 PM
Liver Meridian 1 - 3 AM	Gall Bladder Meridian 11 - 1 AM

Meridian Identification Legend

MERIDIAN	INITIALS
Lung	Lu
Large Intestine	LI
Stomach	St
Spleen	Sp
Heart	Ht
Small Intestine	SI
Bladder	Bl
Kidney	Ki
Pericardium	Pe
Triple Heater	TH
Gall Bladder	GB
Liver	Liv
Conception Vessel	CV
Governing Vessel	GV

Feline Anatomy

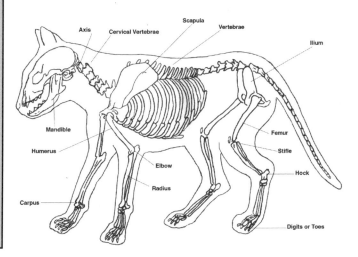

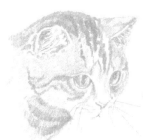

LUNG MERIDIAN
controller of receiving chi

SISTER MERIDIAN - Large Intestine
MAXIMAL TIME - 3 - 5 am
ENERGY - YIN
ELEMENT - Metal

SEASON - Fall
GOVERNED PART OF BODY -
    Skin and Body Hair
COLOR - White or Silver

INDICATORS

PHYSICAL
Respiratory conditions including asthma,
    pneumonia or coughing
Chest pain or congestion
Dry skin or dull coat

BEHAVIOR
Compulsive behaviors
Chronic grief
Depression

FUNCTION

    The Lung Meridian takes in Chi from the air and builds resistance to external intrusions. It regulates the secretion of sweat and skin moistening. It also governs body hair and skin. This meridian eliminates noxious gases through exhalation.

    It is said that the Lung Meridian rules the Chi. The lungs receive Chi, change it and disburse it throughout the entire body. How much or how little Chi is absorbed defines the Chi. For instance shallow breaths display as erratic and often nervous energy while deep breaths create more vitality and grounding. Since air has Chi, as the cat inhales, Chi is brought into his lungs. The outer air Chi in the lungs blends with the Chi from the digestive system and forms what is known as *Gathering Chi*. The Gathering Chi is the life force energy that maintains the animal and its physiological activities. The lungs distribute this essential life force energy throughout the body.

LOCATION

    The Lung Meridian begins internally and surfaces in the hollow of the chest, where it meets the inside of the foreleg, near the underarm in the pectoral muscle. This point is known as Lu 1. The meridian then flows upward at a slight angle, then down to the forearm and runs along the inside edge of the large muscle on the forearm. Then, it flows on the inside edge of the lower leg, ending at the tip of the dewclaw. There are 11 acupoints on the Lung Meridian.

Lung Meridian

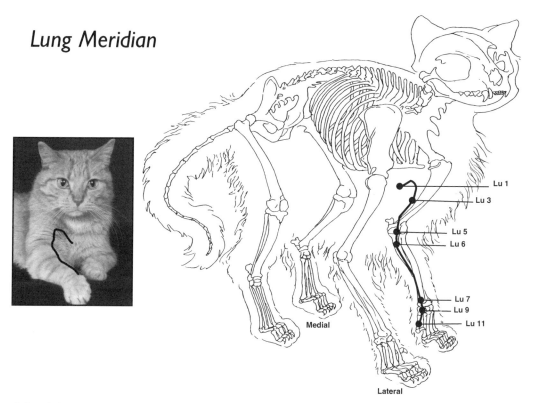

POINT	TYPE OF POINT *Traditional Name*	FUNCTION
Lu 1	Alarm Point for the lung *Central Palace*	Relieves fatigue and strengthens the lungs. Use to treat neck, shoulder or upper back aches. Use for loud coughs or asthma. Relieves stagnant Chi associated with grief or trauma.
Lu 3	*Heavenly Residence*	Use for issues of aloofness or withdrawal. Helps relieve negative behavior patterns and relieves depression.
Lu 5	Sedation Point *Foot Marsh*	Main point for muscular disorders and foreleg pain. Relieves elbow pain.
Lu 7	Connecting Point *Broken Sequence*	Master Point for the head and neck. Use for any respiratory condition. Improves Circulation of Defensive Chi, opens pores and stimulates sweating.
Lu 9	Tonification& Source Point *Great Abyss*	Influential Point for arteries. Relieves breathing difficulties and clears the lungs. Relieves elbow and shoulder pain.
Lu 11	Ting Point *Lesser Metal*	Use for acute emergencies such as respiratory failure or collapse. Strengthens the immune system. Relieves acute severe throat conditions.

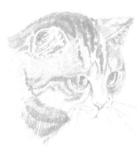

LARGE INTESTINE MERIDIAN
the great eliminator

SISTER MERIDIAN - Lung
MAXIMAL TIME - 5 - 7 am
ENERGY - Yang
ELEMENT - Metal

SEASON - Fall
GOVERNED PART OF BODY -
Skin and Body Hair
COLOR - White or Silver

INDICATORS
PHYSICAL
Constipation or diarrhea
Respiratory conditions
Restricted or tight muscles of the neck
      or shoulder
Skin problems
Weak immune system

BEHAVIOR
Excessive apprehension
Stubbornness

FUNCTION
     The large intestine receives food and water from the small intestine, then absorbs some of the fluids and excretes the remainder. The elimination function of the large intestine has an energetic as well as a physical importance. This meridian helps remove stagnant Chi energy through excretion. Additionally, the Large Intestine Meridian supports the lung in its functions of respiration and immune system activities.

LOCATION
     The Large Intestine Meridian begins at the front inside corner of the foreleg on the medial side of the second toe. From here the meridian flows up on the inside middle of the foreleg. It then crosses laterally over the wrist and flows up on the topside of the foreleg to the elbow up the shoulder and across the ventral portion of the neck. It crosses the mandible and ends at the bottom of the nostril. There are 20 acupoints along this meridian.

Large Intestine Meridian

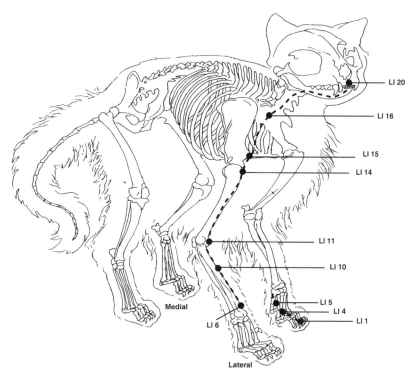

LI 20
LI 16
LI 15
LI 14
LI 11
LI 10
LI 5
LI 4
LI 1
LI 6

Medial

Lateral

POINT	TYPE OF POINT *Traditional Name*	FUNCTION
LI 1	*Metal Yang*	Relieves shoulder pain, shoulder arthritis or toothaches. Benefits acute conjunctivitus. Clears the mind.
LI 4	Source Point *Joining Valley*	Master Point for the face and mouth. Relieves head, neck, foreleg and shoulder pain. Important pain-reducing point, beneficial for pain in any part of the body. Balances the gastrointestinal system. Builds the immune system. Use in conjunction with LI 11. Use to strengthen weak or atrophied muscles.
LI 6	*Slanting Passage*	Connecting Point to the Lung meridian. Relieves throat problems and pain in the wrist and foreleg.
LI 10	*Arm Three Miles*	Use to relieve pain or paralysis of the arm or shoulder. Helps arthritic conditions of the elbow. Builds endurance. Important tonification point.
LI 11	Tonification Point *Crooked Pond*	Relieves diarrhea and benefits the immune system. Relaxes muscular tension and relieves pain. Use for arthritic elbow, acute lower back pain and in the treatment of allergic and infectious disorders.
LI 14	*Upper Arm*	Relieves shoulder tension and relaxes shoulder muscles. Use for relief of stiff neck or eye problems.
LI 15	*Shoulder Bone*	Relieves arthritis of the elbow and shoulder.
LI 20	*Welcome Fragrance*	Use for any nasal problems including sneezing, runny nose, allergies or sinus problems.

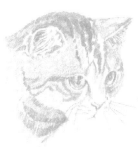

STOMACH MERIDIAN
sea of nourishment

SISTER MERIDIAN - Spleen
MAXIMAL TIME - 7 - 9 am
ENERGY - Yang
ELEMENT - Earth

SEASON - Late Summer
GOVERNED PART OF BODY -
    Muscles & Lymph
COLOR – Yellow

INDICATORS

PHYSICAL

Digestive tract disorders
Eye problems
Stifle problems including
    inflammation, pain and arthritis
Jaw tension and pain
Lethargy and weakness

BEHAVIOR

Chronic nervous tension
Restlessness and anxiety

FUNCTION

The stomach is in charge of digestion. It receives and transforms all food going through the body and assists with its appetite mechanism. The stomach and spleen transport the food essences and Chi to all parts of the body. Stomach Chi and Spleen Chi are responsible for nourishing the muscles. No matter what the disease, it is believed that if the stomach Chi is strong, the outlook is good. Conversely, if the stomach Chi is low, the prognosis is not good.

LOCATION

The Stomach Meridian starts under the eye. This point is St 1. It descends to the nose and travels along the side of the jawbone up to the ear. From here the meridian runs down below the cervical vertebrae through the chest and along the lower edge of the abdomen and loin regions. It then passes over the front aspect of the thigh and stifle, over the tibia and ends at the edge of the third toe. The Stomach Meridian has 45 acupoints.

Stomach Meridian

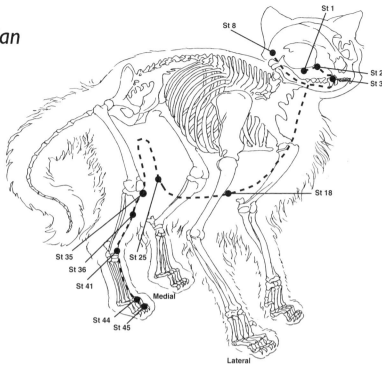

POINT	TYPE OF POINT *Traditional Name*	FUNCTION
St 1	*Receiving Tears*	Use for disorders of the face including eye problems, toothaches, jaw tension and facial paralysis.
St 2	*Four Whites*	Relaxes muscles, tendons and the body in general. Excellent pain relief point. Use for all eye problems.
St 8	*Head Support*	Relieves pain and brightens the eyes. Use for excessive tearing.
St 18	*Breast Root*	Regulates and facilitates lactation.
St 25	Alarm Point for large intestine *Heavenly Pillar*	Use for abdominal disorders and to increase circulation in the legs. Relieves leg pain. Helps relieve diarrhea or constipation and vomiting.
St 35	*Calf's Nose*	Relieves hind leg joint pain. Reduces pain or arthritis of the stifle.
St 36	*Leg Three Miles*	Master Point for the abdomen and gastrointestinal tract. Improves overall strength, health and resistance to disease. Tonifies Chi and harmonizes Defensive Chi. Clears and strengthens the mind. Relieves fatigue. Stimulation of this point benefits digestion and helps restore the immune system. It can be used to increase contractions during labor. Relieves urinary problems.
St 41	Tonification Point *Dispersing Stream*	For lameness of the hind legs, hind limb and joint soreness or abdominal disorders.
St 44	*Inner Courtyard*	Relieves restlessness and anxiety. Use for skin and intestinal disorders. Benefits gingivitis.
St 45	Sedation & Ting Point *Evil's Dissipation*	Relieves indigestion and abdominal pain. Improves circulation and mental clarity.

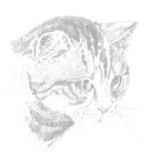

SPLEEN MERIDIAN
controller of distribution

SISTER MERIDIAN - Stomach
MAXIMAL TIME - 9 - 11 am
ENERGY - Yin
ELEMENT - Earth

SEASON - Late Summer
GOVERNED PART OF BODY -
   Muscles & Lymph
COLOR – Yellow

INDICATORS

PHYSICAL
Immune system deficiency or disorders
Muscle problems including atrophy
   lack of tone or strength
Digestive disorders including diarrhea
   and weight problems

BEHAVIOR
Timid or insecure nature
Lack of awareness

FUNCTION
The Spleen organ system is responsible for nourishment, including physical, emotional and mental nourishment. The spleen and the stomach assist the digestive processes by transporting and transforming food, absorbing the nourishment and then separating the useable from the unusable food. The spleen is the primary organ in the production of Prenatal Chi. Ingested food and drink provide Food Chi and is the basis for the creation of Postnatal Chi. The spleen governs blood. The Spleen Meridian supplies the essential body energy for the cat and is the core of the immune system.

The Spleen Meridian also governs the muscles, connective tissue and the four limbs; it both originates and carries Chi to these areas. Proper movement is dependent upon a well-balanced Spleen Meridian.

LOCATION
The Spleen Meridian begins on the medial aspect of the hind leg at a point just inside the second toe. It then proceeds up the inner back side of the lower leg, turns slightly forward passing over the hock, then up the middle of the inside leg along the back of the tibia to the stifle. It continues up the femur, then slants toward the head, running along the underside of the abdomen. It then turns and travels toward the rear of the cat, ending about in the sixth intercostal space, approximately level with the point of the shoulder.

Spleen Meridian

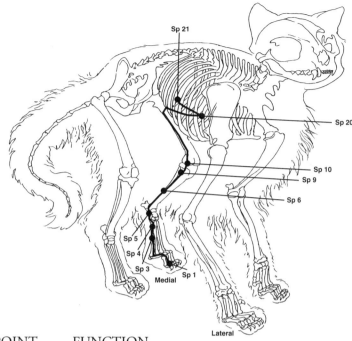

POINT	TYPE OF POINT *Traditional Name*	FUNCTION
Sp 1	Ting Point *Hidden White*	Helps balance energy of the entire meridian. Strengthens the spleen, stops bleeding and regulates the mind.
Sp 3	Source Point *Greater White*	Stimulates poor appetite. Improves skin and muscle tone. Use for chronic back problems. Relieves worry and mental exhaustion. Stabilizes emotions.
Sp 4	Connecting Point *Minute Connecting Channel*	Relieves indigestion with chronic loose stools. Improves circulation of the legs. Relieves nausea, vomiting and diarrhea.
Sp 5	Sedation Point *Gold Mound*	Use for connective tissue weakness and stomach pain.
Sp 6	Master Point for Urogenital Systems *Three Yin Meeting*	Junction of the three Yin channels of spleen, kidney and liver. Good point to work to relieve fatigue or weakness. Relieves gastrointestinal disorders and is effective for relief of chronic diarrhea. Use for allergic or immune-related disorders. Regulates the circulatory and urinary systems. Aids in the relief of pelvic limb problems. Strengthens female reproductive system. Do not use during pregnancy, stimulation can promote labor. Calms the mind, regulates the skin and joints.
Sp 9	*Yin Mound Spring*	Use for skin, arthritic, urinary and reproductive disorders.
Sp 10	*Sea of Blood*	Relieves stifle pain. Builds immune system. Use to relieve female cycle disorders.
Sp 21	*General Control*	General Connecting Point. Relieves muscle pain throughout the body. Helps stop vomiting.

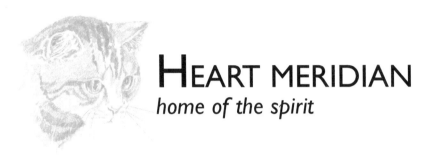

HEART MERIDIAN
home of the spirit

SISTER MERIDIAN - Small Intestine
MAXIMAL TIME - 11 am - 1 pm
ENERGY - Yin
ELEMENT - Fire

SEASON - Summer
GOVERNED PART OF BODY -
  Vascular System
COLOR – Red

INDICATORS
PHYSICAL
Shoulder problems
Restlessness, disturbed sleep
Cardiovascular problems including heart
    irregularities, shortness of breath and
    poor circulation
Nervous system disorders

BEHAVIOR
Hyperactivity
Depression

FUNCTION

The Heart Meridian governs the entire vascular system, controlling the direction and strength of blood flow. It is the center of emotional and mental consciousness and regulates memory and other brain functions. The Heart Meridian encourages good circulation. Good circulation brings nourishment to the tissues, removes toxins and influences all the other organs. Since it rules the mental energy, it is known as Shen, or spirit of an animal. Because of its importance, the heart has a protector, the pericardium. The Pericardium Meridian helps absorb emotional and physical affronts to the cat.

LOCATION

The Heart Meridian begins close to the heart in the armpit. It travels down the foreleg on the inside, crossing behind the wrist and continuing down the back edge on the outside of the foreleg. It ends at a point on the inside tip of the fifth toe. This is the Ting Point, called Ht 9.

Heart
Meridian

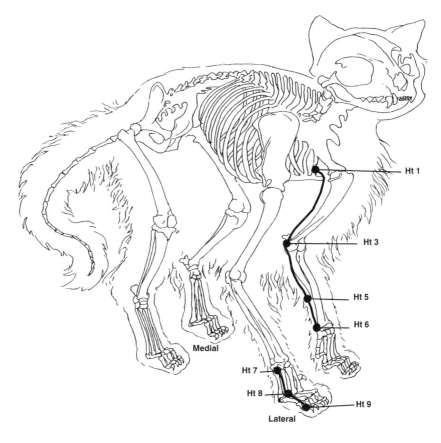

Ht 1

Ht 3

Ht 5

Ht 6

Medial

Ht 7

Ht 8

Ht 9

Lateral

POINT	TYPE OF POINT *Traditional Name*	FUNCTION
Ht 1	*Supreme Spring*	Clears energy flow of the meridian. Relieves arthritis of the shoulder and is useful in relaxing your cat. Relieves depression.
Ht 5	Connecting Point *Inner Communication*	Use to relieve vision disorders. Calms the spirit.
Ht 6	Accumulation Point *Yin Accumulation*	Use for behavioral problems, helps in calming.
Ht 7	Sedation and Source Point *Mind Door*	Important point to balance "disturbances of the spirit." Relieves acute nervous tension and anxiety. Use to calm your cat.
Ht 9	Ting and Tonification Point *Lesser Yin Rushing*	Helps to balance energy of the entire meridian. Use to reduce fever and for cardiovascular emergencies or seizures. Helps relieve anxiety.

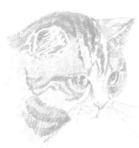

SMALL INTESTINE MERIDIAN
controller of assimilation

SISTER MERIDIAN - Heart
MAXIMAL TIME - 1 - 3 pm
ENERGY - Yang
ELEMENT – Fire

SEASON - Summer
GOVERNED PART OF BODY
   Vascular System
COLOR – Red

INDICATORS

PHYSICAL
Shoulder problems including muscle
   atrophy or stiffness
Foreleg problems
Neck stiffness

BEHAVIOR
Lack of mental clarity
Lack of enthusiasm
Depression

FUNCTION
    The Small Intestine Meridian has a vital function in nourishing the body. It is responsible for receiving and transforming nourishment by absorbing food and drink, separating the pure, useful substances from the impure, waste products. It is also in charge of assimilation of nutrients. On an emotional level, the small intestine rules discernment. It is paired with the Heart Meridian and helps bring clarity of mind.

LOCATION
    The Small Intestine Meridian begins on the fifth toe. Staying on the outside of the leg it travels up, over the metacarpal bones, and reaches back slightly as it goes over the elbow. It flows over the triceps muscle to a point right behind the shoulder joint. From here the meridian flows up the scapula, crossing slightly below its top border and continues up the middle of the neck. It touches the jaw bone and ends at a point on the outside of the base of the ear. There are 19 acupoints along the Small Intestine Meridian.

Small Intestine Meridian

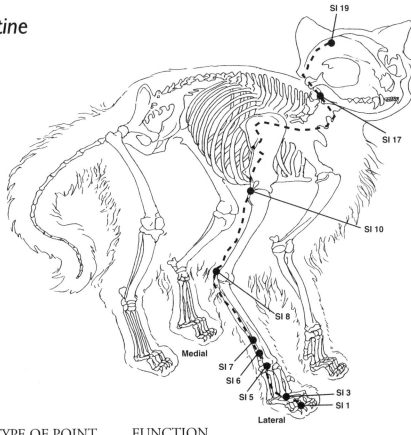

POINT	TYPE OF POINT *Traditional Name*	FUNCTION
SI 1	Ting Point *Lesser Marsh*	Balances entire meridian's energy. Improves lactation.
SI 3	Tonification Point *Back Stream*	Use for arthritis of the ankle, wrist or shoulder pain. Strengthens the spine. Clears the mind and relieves agitation. Relieves acute and chronic neck problems.
SI 5	*Yang Valley*	Use for carpal joint problems. Clears the mind.
SI 6	Accumulation Point *Supporting the Old*	Relieves stiff neck, foreleg, joint or shoulder pain. Benefits the tendons and eyes.
SI 7	Connecting Point *Branch to Heart*	For shoulder, elbow or foreleg problems. Calms the mind.
SI 10	*Scapula's Hollow*	Shoulder release point. Use for generalized spinal stiffness.
SI 17	*Heaven Appearance*	Softens hard muscles and balances the glands.
SI 19	*Listening Palace*	Benefits the ears.

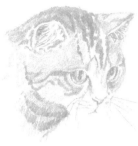

BLADDER MERIDIAN

SISTER MERIDIAN - Kidney
MAXIMAL TIME - 3 - 5 pm
ENERGY - Yang
ELEMENT - Water

SEASON - Winter
BODY PARTS - Bone & Marrow
COLOR - Blue

INDICATORS
PHYSICAL
Urinary tract problems
Lower back and hock problems
General body pain, muscle spasms
    or cramps of the hindquarters
Arthritis, bone or joint problems
Sensitivity in any of the
    Association Points

BEHAVIOR
Fear
Chronic anxiety
Agitation
Depression

FUNCTION
    The bladder transforms fluids through storage and excretion. The Bladder Meridian has the unique capacity of balancing the entire meridian system. Association Points along the Bladder Meridian correspond directly with each of the twelve major meridians. If an Association Point is reactive or tender to the touch, it may indicate an energy imbalance in the corresponding meridian. On an emotional level the lower channel of the Bladder Meridian addresses fear, depression, grief and agitation.

LOCATION
    The Bladder Meridian begins on a point at the inside corner of the cat's eye and runs up and over the top of the head. It flows down the neck and at the shoulders it splits into two branches. The two branches follow lines parallel to the spine. The top channel runs ½ to 1 ½ finger widths off the spine, the second branch runs 1–3 finger widths lower. The channels flow down the back toward the tail and continue down the hind leg. The two channels pass between the crease of the biceps femoris and semitendinosus muscles. The Bladder Meridian then flows down the outside aspect of the hind leg and ends at Bl 67, the Ting Point. This point is on the lateral aspect of the fifth toe.

Bladder Meridian

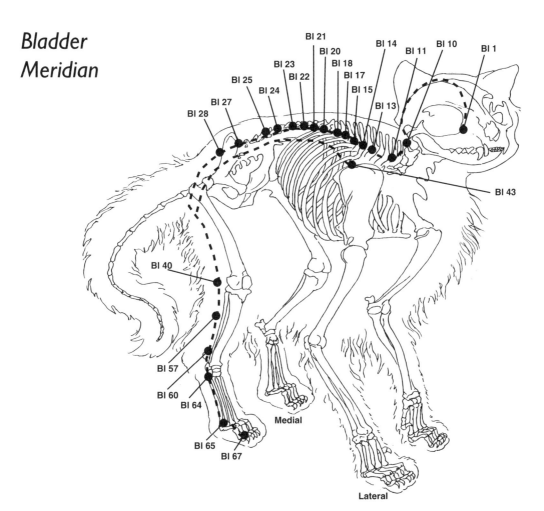

POINT	TYPE OF POINT *Traditional Name*	FUNCTION
Bl 1	*Eye Brightness*	Excellent point for eye problems including glaucoma, conjunctivitis and early-stage cataract. Benefits nasal disorders and problems of the nervous system.
Bl 10	*Heaven Pillar*	This point is a gate to energy flow between the head and body. Use to relieve depression or fear. Benefits the eyes. Use for cervical, shoulder or back pain.
Bl 11	Influential Point for bone *Big Reed*	Use this point for any type of bone or joint disorder. Enhances bone healing. Helps relieves arthritis, joint deformation and neck and spinal stiffness. Tonifies the Blood.

(Continued on next page)

(Bladder Meridian continued)

POINT	TYPE OF POINT *Traditional Name*	FUNCTION
Bl 13	Lung Association Point *Lung Back Transporting Point*	Use for lung problems including bronchitis or asthma.
Bl 14	Pericardium Association Point *Terminal Yin Back*	Calming effect. Regulates the heart.
Bl 15	Heart Association Point *Heart Back Transporting Point*	Calming effect. Stimulates the brain.
Bl 17	*Diaphragm Back Transporting Point*	Nourishes and invigorates the Blood. Calms the mind. Helps relieve vomiting, hiccups and nausea. Relieves skin disorders.
Bl 18	Liver Association Point *Liver Back Transporting Point*	Benefits the liver and gall bladder and eyes.
Bl 20	Spleen Association Point *Spleen Back Transporting Point*	Tonifies the spleen and stomach and nourishes the blood. Reinforce in all chronic diseases and energy depletion.
Bl 21	Stomach Association Point *Stomach Back Transporting Point*	Use for gastrointestinal disorders.
Bl 22	Triple Heater Association Point *Triple Heater Back Transporting Point*	Relieves abdominal pain, hormone problems and lower back pain. Can benefit urinary problems and kidney stones.
Bl 23	Kidney Association Point *Kidney Back Transporting Point*	General arthritis point. Helps relieve chronic lower back and lumbosacral pain. Strengthens the immune system. Helps stabilize Yin – Yang balance. Benefits bones, the spine and joints.
Bl 24	*Sea of Chi*	Use for acute or chronic lumbosacral pain.
Bl 25	Lg Intestine Association Point *Lg Intestine Back Transporting Point*	Helps relieve constipation and diarrhea and abdominal pain and distension. Use for local back pain.
Bl 27	Sm Intestine Association Point *Sm Intestine Back Transporting Point*	Relieves indigestion. Use for abdominal pain, diarrhea, and frequent urination.
Bl 28	Bladder Association Point *Bladder Back Transporting Point*	Helps relieve urinary bladder problems. Use to relieve lower back, sciatica or leg pain.
Bl 40	Master Point for lower back and hips *Supporting Middle*	Point relieves pain or stiffness along the Bladder Meridian in the lower back, hip and stifle areas. Use for skin disorders and itching. Benefits urinary tract infections.

POINT	TYPE OF POINT *Traditional Name*	FUNCTION
Bl 57	*Supporting Mountain*	Relieves cramps of the gastrocnemius muscle and lower back pain. Use for general muscle tension.
Bl 60	*Kunlun Mountain*	Known as the "aspirin" point, it relieves pain throughout the body. Used for chronic back pain. Relieves stiffness of the shoulder, neck and occipital regions.
Bl 64	Source Point *Capital Bone*	Strengthens the back. Benefits the eyes and clears and strengthens the mind.
Bl 65	Sedation Point *Binding Bone*	Relieves neck pain and stiffness. Use for acute cystitis.
Bl 67	Ting and Tonification Point *Reaching Yin*	Balances energy of the entire Bladder Meridian. Improves eyesight and improves mental focus. Use for difficult labor or retained placenta and malposition of fetus.

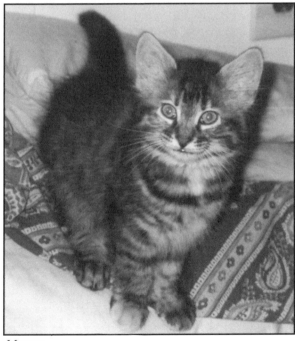

Morgan

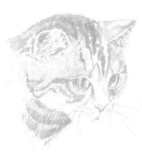

KIDNEY MERIDIAN
residence of resolution

SISTER MERIDIAN - Bladder
MAXIMAL TIME - 5 - 7 pm
ENERGY - Yin
ELEMENT - Water

SEASON - Winter
GOVERNED PART OF BODY -
 Bone & Marrow
COLOR – Blue

INDICATORS

PHYSICAL
Bone problems including fractures
Periodontal diseases
Dull and lifeless coat
Irregular estrous cycles, fertility problems

BEHAVIOR
Fear or timidity
Chronic anxiety
Poor concentration
Aggression

FUNCTION

The Kidney Meridian houses the *Jing* essence, the substance that underlies all organic life. Jing can be likened to a reservoir of energy that nourishes each cell of the body, fuels the metabolism and maintains the vitality, well-being and function of every system. Although Jing is primarily inherited, it can be supplemented and enhanced by a healthy lifestyle including good nutrition, exercise and energy healing work.

The Kidney Meridian controls the growth and healing of bones. Teeth, which are considered in TCM terms to be surplus bone, are also governed by the Kidney Meridian. Since this meridian opens into the ears, proper functioning of the ears depends on a balanced Kidney Meridian. This meridian is responsible for the harmonized sexual functions of your cat.

Emotionally, the Kidney Meridian deals with survival and instinctual fear. A cat who exhibits unusual fear reactions, lacks confidence, or is aggressive will benefit from acupressure work along the Kidney Meridian.

LOCATION

The Kidney Meridian starts at a soft point just under the main foot pad of the hind paw. The meridian travels up the inside of the hind leg to the hock, circles in a clockwise direction, continuing its flow up the inside of the leg to the groin area. It flows along the ventral abdomen, about 2-3 inches off the midline and through the chest, ending at Ki 27, which is located between the breastbone and first rib.

Kidney
Meridian

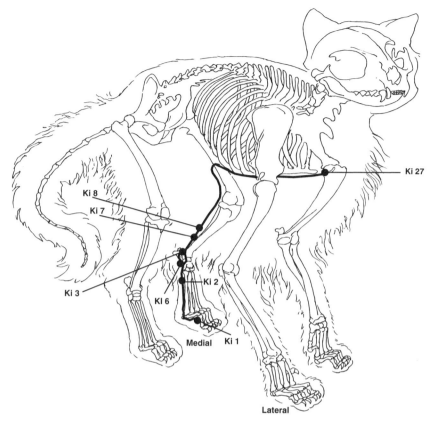

POINT	TYPE OF POINT *Traditional Name*	FUNCTION
Ki 1	Sedation Point *Bubbling Spring*	Use for shock. Reduces aggressive behavior.
Ki 2	*Blazing Valley*	Use for sexual dysfunction.
Ki 3	Source Point *Greater Stream*	Helps restore the immune system. Estrous cycle irregularity. Helps relieve lower back soreness.
Ki 6	*Shining Sea*	Regulates hormones. Releases the shoulders and neck. Calms the mind.
Ki 7	Tonification Point *Returning Current*	Stimulate if your cat is fatigued. Aids in relief of hock and back pain.
Ki 8	*Junction of Faithfulness*	Relieves lower back pain and soreness. Builds confidence.
Ki 27	Association Point for all Association Points *Transporting Point Mansion*	Use for respiratory ailments including asthma or chest pain. Relieves physical and mental tiredness.

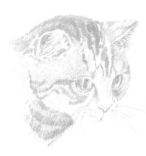

PERICARDIUM MERIDIAN
heart protector

SISTER MERIDIAN - Triple Heater
MAXIMAL TIME - 7 - 9 pm
ENERGY - Yin
ELEMENT - Fire

SEASON - Summer
GOVERNED PART OF BODY -
   Vascular System
COLOR – Red

INDICATORS

PHYSICAL
Stiffness of the neck, foreleg and elbow
Chest conditions including pneumonia
Irregular heart rhythm including
   abnormally rapid heartbeat,
   heart murmurs

BEHAVIOR
Timid behavior
Depression

FUNCTION

The Pericardium Meridian's main function is to protect the heart from external stresses. This protection manifests on both physical and emotional levels. The Pericardium Meridian supports the heart in circulatory functions. Physically this meridian protects the heart by absorbing heat. Emotionally its purpose is to bring joy and protect the heart from emotional stress. The pericardium accomplishes this by balancing the emotions and calming the heart.

LOCATION

The Pericardium Meridian begins deep within the body at the sac that surrounds the heart. The meridian surfaces in the space between the 5th and 6th ribs, near the elbow. From here it travels down the middle of the inside of the foreleg toward the back side of the wrist. Then it runs down the back inside of the lower leg and ends at the tip of the third toe, Pe 9, the Ting Point.

Pericardium Meridian

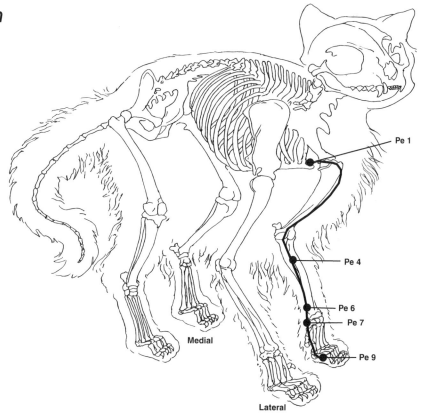

Pe 1

Pe 4

Pe 6

Pe 7

Pe 9

Medial

Lateral

POINT	TYPE OF POINT *Traditional Name*	FUNCTION
Pe 1	*Heavenly Pond*	Use to calm heart palpitations and heart murmurs. Helps with respiratory problems.
Pe 4	*Cleft Door*	Accumulation Point. Calms the heart and relieves fear.
Pe 6	Connecting Point *Inner Gate*	Master Point for chest and cranial abdomen (front of abdomen). Powerful point for all chest conditions including pneumonia. Improves circulation. Powerful anxiety reducer. Balances the internal organs.
Pe 7	Sedation & Source Point *Great Hill*	Calms the spirit and regulates the heart. Use for local wrist or paw problems. Helps relieve skin problems of heat and intense itching.
Pe 9	Ting Point & Tonification Point *Center Rush*	Balances energy of entire meridian. Use for foreleg arthritis. Use for shock and to assist post-operative recovery.

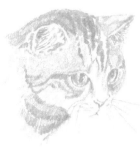

TRIPLE HEATER MERIDIAN
commander of all energies

SISTER MERIDIAN - Pericardium
MAXIMAL TIME - 9 - 11 pm
ENERGY - Yang
ELEMENT - Fire

SEASON - Summer
GOVERNED PART OF BODY -
Vascular System
COLOR – Red

INDICATORS
PHYSICAL
Ear problems
Neck stiffness, tension or pain
Foreleg, shoulder or elbow problems

BEHAVIOR
None

FUNCTION
The Triple Heater is a function rather than a physical organ. It represents a group of energies and involves many organs. This meridian is the functional relationship between the energy-transforming organs. The Triple Heater transforms and transports Chi as it flows unimpeded to all parts of the body. In this role, it helps to excrete waste as well as direct Chi to the organs. This meridian also enhances the function of the lymphatic system.

LOCATION
The Triple Heater Meridian starts at a point on the lateral border of the fourth toe. It flows up the metacarpals and continues up the outside of the upper foreleg. The meridian travels to the elbow, then along the back side of the humerus to the shoulder joint. From here it crosses the scapula and continues up the neck, below the vertebrae to the ear and ends on the outside border of the eye. There are 23 acupoints along the Triple Heater Meridian.

Triple Heater Meridian

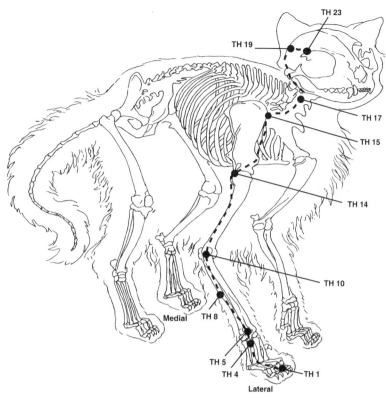

POINT	TYPE OF POINT *Traditional Name*	FUNCTION
TH 1	Ting Point *Gate Rush*	Benefits the eyes and ears. Use for conjunctivitus. Restores consciousness and relieves convulsions.
TH 4	Source Point *Yang's Pond*	Relieves discomfort such as tendinitis, rheumatism, foreleg edema and arthritis. Relaxes the tendons. Use in chronic disease conditions when energy of the kidneys is deficient.
TH 5	Connecting Point *Outer Gate*	For arthritis of the wrist, elbow or shoulder. Helps ease tendinitis and builds the immune system. Relieves ear problems and tense muscles.
TH 8	*Connecting 3 Yang*	Crossing point of the three Yang foreleg meridians, the Small Intestine, Triple Heater and Large Intestine. This is a shoulder, neck and foreleg release point. Benefits the ears.
TH 10	Sedation Point *Heavenly Well*	For elbow and forelimb soreness, sprains and rheumatic pain. Relaxes tendons. Relieves throat and lymph gland problems.
TH 14	*Shoulder Crevice*	Use for shoulder soreness.
TH 15	*Heavenly Crevice*	Important local point for shoulder problems.
TH 17	*Wind Screen*	Use for ear problems.
TH 23	*Silk Bamboo Hole*	Benefits the eyes, relieves pain. Use for conjunctivitus.

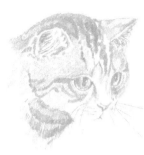

GALL BLADDER MERIDIAN
official of decision and judgment

SISTER MERIDIAN - Liver
MAXIMAL TIME - 11 pm - 1 am
ENERGY - Yang
ELEMENT - Wood

SEASON - Spring
GOVERNED PART OF BODY -
   Ligaments and Tendons
COLOR – Green

INDICATORS

PHYSICAL
Arthritis-joint stiffness or pain
Muscle stiffness, soreness
Ear and eye problems

BEHAVIOR
Anger or aggression
Depression
Timidity and indecision

FUNCTION

   The Gall Bladder Meridian impacts certain aspects of the emotional and energetic properties of your cat. It regulates the flow of Chi throughout the body and governs the decision-making process. Excessive gall bladder Chi may be exhibited as anger, whereas timidity or depression may be a result of insufficient gall bladder Chi. Also, the Gall Bladder Meridian rules many parts of your cat's body including the eyes, ligaments, tendons, and joints.

LOCATION

   The Gall Bladder Meridian begins at the outer corner of the eye. It flows to the outer side of the ear, crossing back and forth on the side of the head. It curves behind the ear and flows down the neck to the middle of the scapula where it enters the chest cavity and flows through the abdomen to GB 24. It travels up to GB 25, a point on the outside of the last rib. The meridian then runs farther up to the pelvic area, below the point of the hip to the hip joint. From here it passes over the femur and down the outside of the hind leg. GB 44, the Ting Point, is the last point on this meridian.

Gall Bladder Meridian

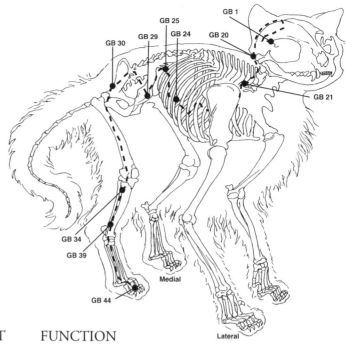

POINT	TYPE OF POINT *Traditional Name*	FUNCTION
GB 1	*Pupil Crevice*	Benefits the eyes. Use for red, sore eyes or conjunctivitus.
GB 20	*Wind Pond*	Alleviates head and neck tension and pain. Helps with eye, ear and nose problems. Nourishes the brain, improves memory. Use for generalized muscular aches.
GB 21	*Shoulder Well*	Relieves shoulder pain and arthritis. Benefits lactation. Softens tense muscles.
GB 24	Alarm Point for the gall bladder *Sun and Moon*	Use to relieve stomach indigestion and disorders, abdominal pain and muscle soreness. Helps remove gallstones.
GB 25	Alarm Point for the kidney *Capital Door*	For kidney disorders and lower back pain.
GB 29	*Squatting Crevice*	Use for joint disorders, especially of the hips.
GB 30	*Jumping Circle*	For hip soreness or dysplasia and sciatica problems. Relaxes the tendons and restores joint mobility. Benefits atrophied leg muscles.
GB 34	*Yang Hill Mound*	Influential Point for the muscles and tendons, use to strengthen weak muscles and relax muscle spasms. Relieves joint stiffness especially of the hips, legs and knees. Regulates the intestines and the Gall Bladder Meridian.
GB 39	*Hanging Bell*	Influential Point for building bone marrow. Tonifies Kidney Jing. Use for weak or spasming muscles. Weakness, stiffness and inflammation of the joints, for bone degeneration. Improves hearing and strengthens the immune system.
GB 44	Ting Point *Orifice Yin*	Helps relieve arthritis and hock problems. Influences the eyes, relieves pain and swelling. Calms the mind.

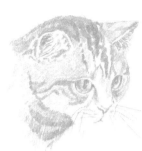

LIVER MERIDIAN
controller of strategic planning

SISTER MERIDIAN - Gall Bladder
MAXIMAL TIME - 1 - 3 am
ENERGY - Yin
ELEMENT - Wood

SEASON - Spring
GOVERNED PART OF BODY -
  Tendons and Ligaments
COLOR – Green

INDICATORS

PHYSICAL
Eye/vision problems
Estrous cycle problems
Digestive problems
Joint Problems
Tendon and ligament problems

BEHAVIOR
Aggressiveness or anger

FUNCTION

The Liver Meridian maintains even and harmonious movement of Chi throughout the body. It is the principal center of metabolism. The Liver Meridian controls hundreds of functions including synthesizing proteins, neutralizing poisons, assisting in the regulation of blood sugar levels and secreting bile. It also governs the flow of Chi in several ways: coordinating digestion and estrous cycles, and harmonizing the emotions. In traditional terms, the Liver Meridian is known as the Controller of Strategic Planning.

A balanced Liver Meridian allows both cat and human to use energy efficiently. The parts of the body related to the Liver Meridian are the tendons and ligaments.

LOCATION

The Liver Meridian begins at a point on the first toe. This point is the Ting Point, Liv 1. The meridian travels up the inside middle of the hind leg, over the hock and up the femur. The meridian enters the groin region and travels toward the front of the cat. Liv 13 is located at the end of the next to the last rib. The meridian then slants down and ends with Liv 14.

Liver
Meridian

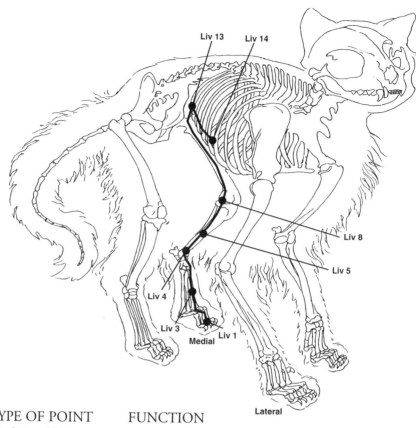

POINT	TYPE OF POINT *Traditional Name*	FUNCTION
Liv 1	Ting Point *Big Thick*	Emergency point, use to restore consciousness. Regulates reproductive cycles. Benefits difficult urination and improves muscle tone to aid urinary incontinence.
Liv 3	Source Point *Bigger Rushing*	Invigorates and clears the meridian system. Provides a generalized calming effect. Benefits vision, improves lactation, circulation and benefits weak muscles.
Liv 4	*Middle Seal*	Helps eye problems. Calming point. Relieves pain in lower abdomen. Use for urinary disorders.
Liv 5	Connecting Point *Gourd Ditch*	Helps resolve reproductive disorders. Relieves emotional tension.
Liv 8	Tonification Point *Spring and Bend*	Relieves stifle problems. Benefits the urinary tract.
Liv 14	Alarm Point for the liver *Cyclic Gate*	Helps with liver problems. Use for muscle soreness.

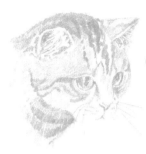

CONCEPTION VESSEL MERIDIAN
controller of strategic planning

SISTER MERIDIAN - None
ENERGY - Yin
AREAS OF INFLUENCE - Abdomen, Thorax, Lungs, Throat and Face

INDICATORS

PHYSICAL
Genital disorders
Problems of the lungs and chest
Reproductive system ailments
Head and neck pain
Itching
Abdominal pain

BEHAVIOR
Anxiety
Hyperactivity

FUNCTION

The Conception Vessel Meridian affects your cat's energy and is responsible for controlling the Yin energy of an animal. It moves stagnant Chi while also regulating the storage and distribution of Jing throughout the body. Therefore, points along its pathway can be used to benefit problems of conception, physical, mental and sexual development, and premature aging. The Conception Vessel absorbs overflow energy from one meridian and redirects it to deficient meridians, thus balancing the energy throughout the body. Aditionally, the Conception Vessel impacts all reproductive functions.

LOCATION

The Conception Vessel Meridian travels the full length of the ventral midline on the cat's body. The meridian begins at a point below the anus (CV 1). It runs between the hind legs, through the genitals and umbilicus, continuing along the midline of the abdomen and through the chest. It then passes up the midline of the neck and ends at a point on the lower lip known as CV 24.

Note: This meridian does not have a sister meridian.

Conception Vessel Meridian

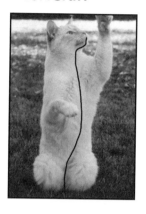

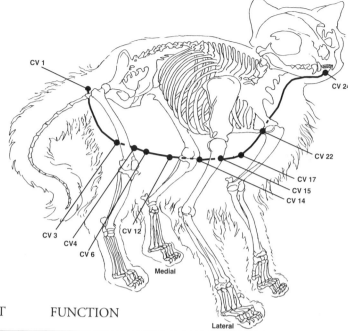

CV 1

CV 24

CV 22

CV 17

CV 15

CV 14

CV 3

CV 12

CV4

CV 6

Medial

Lateral

POINT	TYPE OF POINT *Traditional Name*	FUNCTION
CV 1	*Meeting of Yin*	Use for urogenital problems. Can restore consciousness. Nourishes Yin energy.
CV 3	Alarm Point for the bladder *Middle Extremity*	Meeting of the three Yin meridians: Spleen, Kidney and Liver. Reproduction energy center of the body. Use to relieve incontinence.
CV4	Alarm Point for small intestine *Gate to the Original Chi*	Energy center of the body that stores and distributes Chi and Jing. Benefits reproductive disorders, helps urogenital problems. Regulates the uterus. Benefits ageing issues of poor hearing, vision and weak joints and muscles. Powerful calming point. Use for chronic disorders.
CV 6	*Sea of Chi*	Energy center of the body responsible for energy storage and distribution. Use for a tired, lethargic or depressed cat. Relieves lower abdominal pain and constipation.
CV 12	*Middle of Epigastrium*	Influential Point for all Yang organs. Harmonizes the stomach, relieves gastrointestinal problems and relieves stress. Reduces heart irregularity and stomach stress. Helpful in dealing with behavioral problems.
CV 14	Alarm Point for the heart *Great Palace*	Calms the spirit and mind. Aids nervous anxiety.
CV 15	*Dove Tail*	Source Point of all Yin organs and Connecting Point of Conception Vessel. Powerful calming action for anxiety and emotional upsets.
CV 17	Alarm Point for pericardium *Middle of Chest*	Influential Point for Chi, use to disperse stagnant Chi and improve the overall energy of your cat. Stimulation of this point will increase or disperse energy, depending on your cat's current needs. Use for all lung conditions, especially chronic problems.
CV 22	*Heaven's Projection*	Strengthens the brain and regulates the lungs and throat. Effective for respiratory problems.
CV 24	*Saliva Receiver*	Crossing point of the Conception, Stomach and Large Intestine Meridians. Helps relieve fear and anxiety. Benefits the mouth and face and relieves excessive salivation, mouth and tongue ulcers, gingivitis and tooth pain.

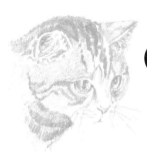

GOVERNING VESSEL MERIDIAN
vessel gathering the yang

SISTER MERIDIAN - None
ENERGY - Yang
AREAS OF INFLUENCE - Head, Back, Spine, Back of Neck

INDICATORS

PHYSICAL
Spinal problems, backache
Nervous disorders
Immune stimulation

BEHAVIOR
Hyperactivity

FUNCTION

The Governing Vessel Meridian helps strengthen the back and spine. It also controls the bladder and assists in coordinating and harmonizing all the organs and regions of the cat's body. The Governing Vessel is said to regulate the central nervous system including the brain, spinal cord and the spinal vertebrae. Like the Conception Vessel, the Governing Vessel acts to redistribute and balance the body's Chi, particularly the Yang aspect of the Chi energy.

LOCATION

The Governing Vessel begins at the depression between the anus and the root of the tail, known as GV 1. The meridian travels along the dorsal midline of the back. It runs over the top of the head and face and ends at GV 26, a point between the upper lip and gums.

Note: This meridian does not have a sister meridian, it runs along a single pathway on the body.

Governing Vessel Meridian

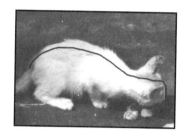

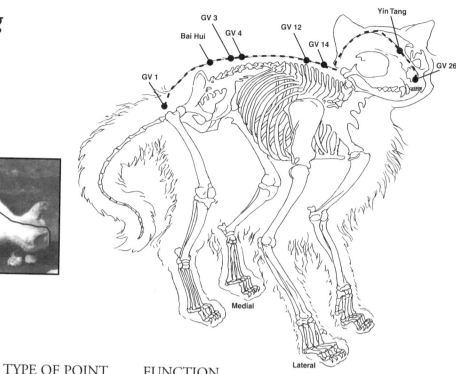

POINT	TYPE OF POINT *Traditional Name*	FUNCTION
GV 1	*Long Strength*	From this point energy circulates up the spine to the head and therefore this point can benefit the spine as well as mental or behavior issues. Use for spinal pain, stiffness spasm or convulsions. Benefits nervous anxiety. Use for constipation and diarrhea. Can stimulate first defecation in newborn kittens.
GV 3	*Lumbar Yang Gate*	Strengthens the lower back and legs.
GV 4	*Gate of Life*	Use to tonify Jing, Chi, and Yang. Relieves intestinal problems and strengthens the urogenital system. Strengthens the lower back and spine.
GV 12	*Body Pillar*	Strengthens the body and lungs. Use after a chronic illness. Relieves lower back pain, stiffness or spasms.
GV 14	*Big Vertebra*	Meeting point of the six Yang meridians. Use for spinal problems involving the neck, shoulders and forelegs. Immuno-stimulation point. Clears the mind.
GV 26	*Middle of Person*	Use for specific emergencies including shock, collapse, heatstroke, seizures or respiratory stimulation in newborns. Benefits the lumbar spine.
GV Yin Tang		Powerful calming point.
Bai Hui		Use for any hindquarter problem, heatstroke or over exertion.

NOTES

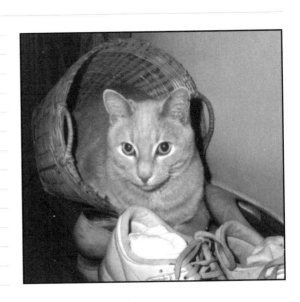

chapter five

Feline Acupressure Points

People who love cats are usually passionate about cats. We take absolute pleasure in watching our cats walk, play, drink water, anything, because we consider them wondrous animals. Caring for cats brings us many blessings. Their gentle souls remind us who we are. Just touching a cat connects us with the better part of ourselves. When caring for their needs, we are also caring for our own needs. We get so caught up in our work, doing household chores and a "catrillion" other things, we forget about the simple joys of life until a fluffy kitty catches our attention. The instant we connect with a cat our whole being changes. We soften inside and feel an inner contentment by just sharing a moment or two with a special feline.

For most of us it is hard to imagine how or why anyone on earth could abandon, neglect or abuse a cat. According to the National Council on Pet Population Study and Policy reported in the Journal of Applied Animal Welfare Science (July 1998), the top five reasons people relinquish cats to shelters are: (1) Moving, (2) Landlord not allowing pets, (3) Too many animals in the household, (4) Cost of pet maintenance, (5) "Owner" having personal problems. Fortunately, in Europe and North America, hundreds of humane shelters do their best to care for unwanted animals. Unfortunately, there is no way they can take care of all of the animals arriving on their door steps.

The Humane Society of the United States (HSUS) spaying and neutering campaign has shown some success; shelter populations are generally down and adoptions are up. But we still have a long way to go before we can consider our communities humane and caring places. A 1992 HSUS survey found that 25% of American households feed stray cats. Another interesting, though sad, statistic is that feral cats (domesticated cats who have reverted to be wild) have harsh, brief lives. During their two-to-three year life span, a feral cat is constantly hungry, females are consistently pregnant, and only 33% of kittens are still alive at one year. These facts punctuate how far we have yet to go to repay the debt we owe our feline friends for sharing their lives with us.

The smallest feline is a masterpiece.
– Leonardo da Vinci

Acupressure, human caring, and cats are a good combination for mending the most torn people and cats. We have seen acupressure and other forms of natural healing make a big difference in many lives. We hope you will be one of the hundreds to contribute your healing abilities to your community. Learning the acupressure points, more commonly referred to as acupoints, is the next step to becoming a student of caring for cats through acupressure.

Acupoints

Acupoint work is the core of an acupressure treatment. An acupoint is the specific place along a meridian where Chi energy flows. At these particular sites, which are often near the surface of the cat's body, Chi is accessible to manipulation. Acupoints can be viewed as pools of energy that, when stimulated, improve the flow of Chi along a meridian. Although the specific acupoint is between the size of the point of a needle and a green pea, the area of effectiveness is thought to be the size of a dime or penny.

Usually acupoints are located in the valleys of the body, not on a bony prominence or in the belly of a muscle. You find them in the depressions next to or between muscles and bones, and around joints. For their small size a healthy cat is surprisingly strong. Just try to make them do something they don't want and you will know how strong cats really are. It is easy to distinguish bone from muscle on a strong, lean cat, though the length and density of fur may make finding an acupoint quite tricky.

While you are learning the meridians, feel for the lines between muscle and bone with your index and middle fingers. Become aware of the different sensations on your cat's body. Let your finger rest on places that feel warm or cool, dense or soft, depressed or protruding. Acupressure requires educated hands combined with intuition and healing intent.

Acupoints are usually located in the valleys of the body, not on a bony prominence or in the belly of a muscle. You find them in the depressions next to or between muscles and bones, and around joints.

The purpose of performing point work is two-fold: the first is to locate the potential imbalances in the meridian network and the second is to work with the points that will restore balance and harmony in the cat's body. An acupoint either can have excessive or deficient Chi energy. Using acupoint techniques, the practitioner releases energy that has become blocked, congested, or stagnant along the meridian. To bring Chi to a deficient area, you need to strengthen or tonify the acupoint. To reduce excessive Chi, you sedate the appropriate acupoint to disperse the energy.

Each of the twelve major meridians and the two Extraordinary Vessels have acupoints that TCM practitioners consider either as permanent or interim acupoints. Interim points appear during states of illness or injury and may or may not be located on a meridian pathway. Permanent acupoints exist at all times and are identified by their functions, locations, and effects. The charts in this chapter refer only to the permanent acupoints.

Acupoints are classified by their functions, benefits, and information they provide when their specific characteristics are interpreted. Knowing and understanding how to use the different point categories during an acupressure treatment is a powerful tool.

Certain acupoints have particular beneficial properties. These acupoints are grouped together under a single classification determined by the benefit these points provide. For instance, when the Master Point for the back and hips is included in a treatment for a cat

If a man could be crossed with the cat, it would improve the man but deteriorate the cat.
– Mark Twain

with a broken hind leg, working this point can significantly enhance the impact of the treatment. Because sister meridians are a reflection of each other, working with

A chart is a general guide for locating acupoints - not an absolute one. Relax, feel the energy, and use your intuition to locate acupoints. Often acupoints look different, feel harder or softer, and are more sensitive to the touch than the surrounding area or remainder of the meridian pathway.

the Connecting Points on one meridian can short circuit an imbalance of Chi on the sister meridian, initiating a return to harmony.

Other categories of acupoints provide the practitioner with valuable information about the cat's condition. Each organ system has an associated point within the grouping of Association Points located along the Bladder Meridian. If an Association Point is sensitive to the touch then you know there is an imbalance along the meridian represented. If your cat demonstrates a sensitivity to Bladder 15 (BL 15) when you touch the acupoint lightly, it may indicate an acute condition along the associated Heart Meridian. Since blockages along the Heart Meridian often involve emotions and Shen Chi, have you observed any changes in your cat's attitudes or behavior? Does your cat seem more fearful or guarded than usual? Does his body seem stiffer lately? Is he less active? Does he seem depressed or worried? Have you made any changes in your cat's environment that may be stressful for your feline friend?

Understanding the basic nature of each of the groupings of points and being familiar with the types of conditions they each indicate will help you in performing an acupressure treatment. For example, knowing that the Accumulation Point Lung 6 (Lu 6) can help sedate or disperse a painfully acute respiratory condition will give you a greater amount of knowledge and sense of confidence when working with your cat.

The descriptions and charts identifying the acupoint classifications are on the remaining pages of this chapter. For detailed descriptions of acupressure Point Work technique and further information about characteristics of acupoints refer to Chapter Three, Feline Acupressure Treatment.

Transpositional Versus Traditional Points

There is an ongoing debate regarding the exact location of acupoints. The two schools of thought are: Traditional and Transpositional.

The Traditional school identifies points used on animals in China for over four thousand years. The use of these points is based on the acupoints' effects and are not necessarily associated with a meridian.

The Transpositional school recognizes points taken from the human meridian system and anatomically transposes the points to animals. The meridian pathways offer a guide or approximation to the location of acupoints, although some anatomical differences must be accommodated.

We have consistently used Transpositional points in our practice, training, and publications. We have found them to be an abundant resource for promoting healing. This debate is apt to carry on for many more years, but the real test is the results we achieve with our cats. We encourage you to feel the energy in your cat's body and let your educated intuition guide you in your healing work.

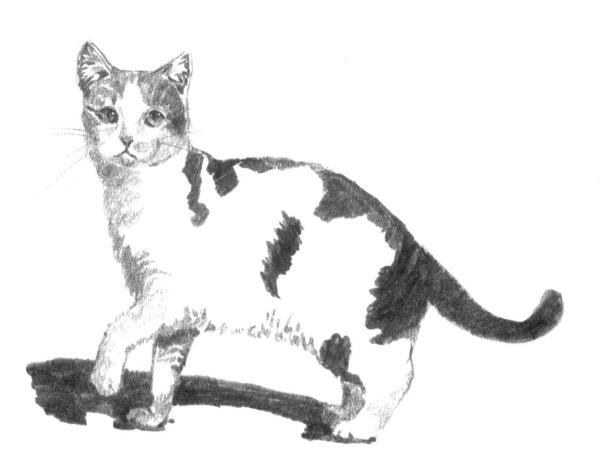

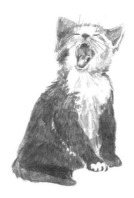

ACCUMULATION POINTS

Definition

    The Accumulation Points are where the Chi energy actually accumulates. In China the Accumulation Points are called "hung" points; the word hung means great temples. The Accumulation Points are as spiritually and physically significant to the health and balance of the body as the great temples are to human life.

Benefit

    Accumulation Points are where the Chi of the meridian gathers. These points are used primarily in acute conditions, especially if pain is present. Usually these points need to be sedated. Treating the Accumulation Points removes obstructions by dispersing energy and rebalancing the flow of Chi along the meridian. A beneficial property of all Accumulation Points is that they can help stop bleeding and relieve pain along their meridian pathway. Accumulation points are usually used in combination with other points.

Location

    The Accumulation Points are located from the paw to the elbow on the foreleg and from the paw to the stifle on the hind leg. There is one exception, St 34, which is located just above the stifle.

Accumulation Points

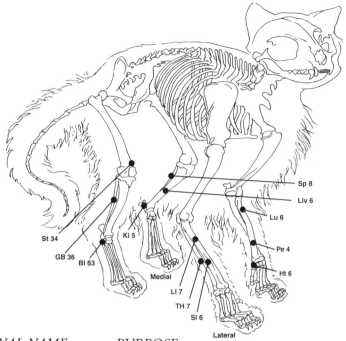

St 34
GB 36 Bl 63
Ki 5
Medial
LI 7
TH 7
SI 6
Lateral
Sp 8
Liv 6
Lu 6
Pe 4
Ht 6

POINTS	*TRADITIONAL NAME*	PURPOSE
Lu 6	*Biggest Hole*	Use for acute, severe respiratory conditions including asthma.
LI 7	*Warm Flow*	Relieves pain of rheumatism and tendinitis of the forelimb. Helps relieve acute conditions along the Large Intestine Meridian. Often used with LI 4.
St 34	*Beam Mound*	Helps relieve acute, painful conditions of the stifle. Also used for acute stomach disorders like vomiting nausea or gastritis.
Sp 8	*Earth Pivot*	Regulates the uterus, moves and relieves pain of the lower abdomen and legs.
Ht 6	*Yin Accumulation*	Relieves pain along the forelimb and is a calming point. Tonifies Heart Yin.
SI 6	*Nourishing the Old*	Relieves acute elbow, shoulder or neck pain. Benefits the tendons and eyes.
Bl 63	*Golden Door*	Use for acute urinary problems, pain along the Bladder Meridian, acute cystitis and acute abdominal pain.
Ki 5	*Water Spring*	Regulates the uterus, benefits urination and relieves abdominal pain.
Pe 4	*Cleft Door*	Calms the heart and regulates its rhythm. Excellent pain relief and calming point.
TH 7	*Converging Channels*	Relieves neck, shoulder or elbow pain. Benefits the eyes and ears.
GB 36	*Outer Mound*	Relieves stiffness, cramps or weakness of hind limbs. Relieves stifle pain.
Liv 6	*Middle Capital*	Relieves pain and obstructions along entire meridian. Relieves acute cystitis.

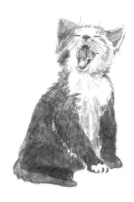

ALARM POINTS

Definition
Each of the Yin/Yang organs has an Alarm Point located on the ventral aspect of the cat's trunk. Energy of the organ gathers at these points. The Alarm Points received their name because they may indicate an organ involvement or energy imbalance when they are tender to the touch. There is one Alarm Point that directly corresponds to each organ or meridian.

Benefit
Practitioners use the Alarm Points in conjunction with the Association Points to differentiate between a meridian blockage or possible organ involvement. Sensitivity to both the Association Point and Alarm Point indicates a possible organ or organ and meridian problem. Sensitivity to the Association Point alone indicates a problem along that meridian's pathway and no organ involvement. Check the Alarm Points and if one is found to be tender further examine the corresponding organ meridian. There are only three Alarm Points located on the meridian for which they are named; they are the Lung, Gall Bladder and Liver Alarm Points. These three organ meridian flows follow each other in the circulation of energy throughout a 24-hour period.

Location
The Alarm Points are located on the ventral chest and abdomen, on the Yin side of the cat's body.

Alarm Points

POINTS	TRADITIONAL NAME	ALARM POINT FOR
Lu 1	*Central Resistance*	Lung
St 25	*Heavenly Pillar*	Large Intestine
CV 12	*Middle of Epigastrium*	Stomach
Liv 13	*Chapter Gate*	Spleen
CV 14	*Great Palace*	Heart
CV 4	*Gate to Original Chi*	Small Intestine
CV 3	*Middle Extremity*	Bladder
GB 25	*Capital Door*	Kidney
CV 17	*Middle of Chest*	Pericardium
CV 5	*Stone Door*	Triple Heater
GB 24	*Sun and Moon*	Gall Bladder
Liv 14	*Cyclic Gate*	Liver

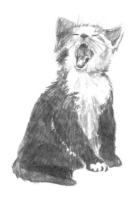

ASSOCIATION POINTS

Definition

The Association or "Back Shu" Points correspond or are "associated" with specific organ meridians. The points are named for their related organs. They offer valuable information, "indicator" data, helping to identify where the imbalance resides and if the imbalance is acute or chronic. They are also used therapeutically.

> The Association Points are also called Back-Shu Points. Shu means to transport. These points transport Chi directly to the organs.

Benefit

The importance of the Association Points in acupressure cannot be overemphasized. They provide a valuable indication system for gathering information about energy imbalances. Overall, the Association Points help balance and regulate the flow of Chi energy throughout your cat's body. These points affect the organs directly and are mostly used to tonify, bringing energy to the organs.

Association Points help to balance your cat's physical and emotional energy. These points also benefit the tissue and sense organ associated with each organ system. As an example, Bl 18 can impact physiological problems of the Liver, such as digestive or reproductive problems as well as the emotional conditions of aggression or anger. At the same time, problems with muscles, the associated tissue and the eyes, the associated sense organ are also benefiting from this Point Work. Because of these properties, it is beneficial for your cat to have the Association Points stimulated during most acupressure treatments. As outlined in the Alarm Points Benefit section, the Association Points, in connection with the Alarm Points help to determine whether there is a meridian imbalance or possible organ involvement.

Location

The twelve Association Points are located along the inner branch of the Bladder meridian between the shoulders and the tail of your cat. They lie on the Bladder meridian approximately ½ to 1½ finger widths on either side of the dorsal midline, lateral to the spinous processes.

Association Points

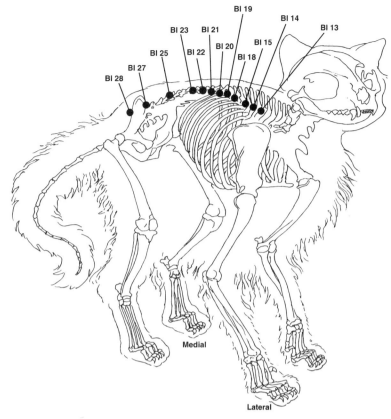

POINTS	*TRADITIONAL NAME*	MERIDIAN
Bl 13	*Lung Back Transporting*	Lung
Bl 14	*Terminal Yin Back Transporting*	Pericardium
Bl 15	*Heart Back Transporting*	Heart
Bl 18	*Liver Back Transporting*	Liver
Bl 19	*Gall Bladder Back Transporting*	Gall Bladder
Bl 20	*Spleen Back Transporting*	Spleen
Bl 21	*Stomach Back Transporting*	Stomach
Bl 22	*Triple Heater Back Transporting*	Triple Heater
Bl 23	*Kidney Back Transporting*	Kidney
Bl 25	*Large Intestine Back Transporting*	Large Intestine
Bl 27	*Small Intestine Back Transporting*	Small Intestine
Bl 28	*Bladder Back Transporting*	Bladder

Note: Association Points are located approximately ½ to 1½ finger widths off the spine.

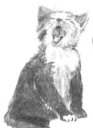

COMMAND POINTS

Metal Points

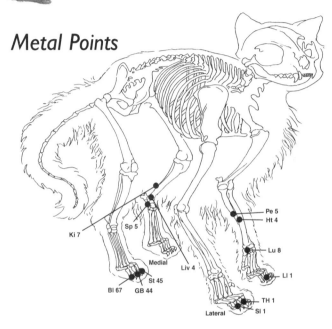

Ki 7
Sp 5
Medial
Liv 4
St 45
Bl 67   GB 44
Lateral

Pe 5
Ht 4
Lu 8
LI 1
TH 1
SI 1

Water Points

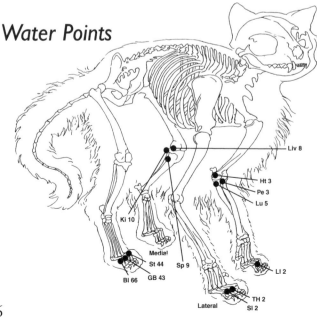

Ki 10
Medial
St 44   Sp 9
Bl 66   GB 43
Lateral

Liv 8
Ht 3
Pe 3
Lu 5
LI 2
TH 2
SI 2

Definition

The Command Points correspond to the points of the five elements in the Five Phases of Transformation: Metal, Water, Wood, Fire and Earth. Each of the twelve meridians has five Command Points, one for each element. Therefore, there are 60 Command Points in total. These are evenly divided into 30 Yin points and 30 Yang points.

Benefit

Points are selected for stimulation based upon either the Control or Creation Cycle of the Five Phases of Transformation and the presenting problem of the cat. See Chapter Two, Traditional Chinese Medicine, for further information. Many practitioners use Command Points as their primary points in an acupressure treatment.

Location

All 60 Command Points are located on the cat's front and hind legs between the foot and elbow and the foot and stifle.

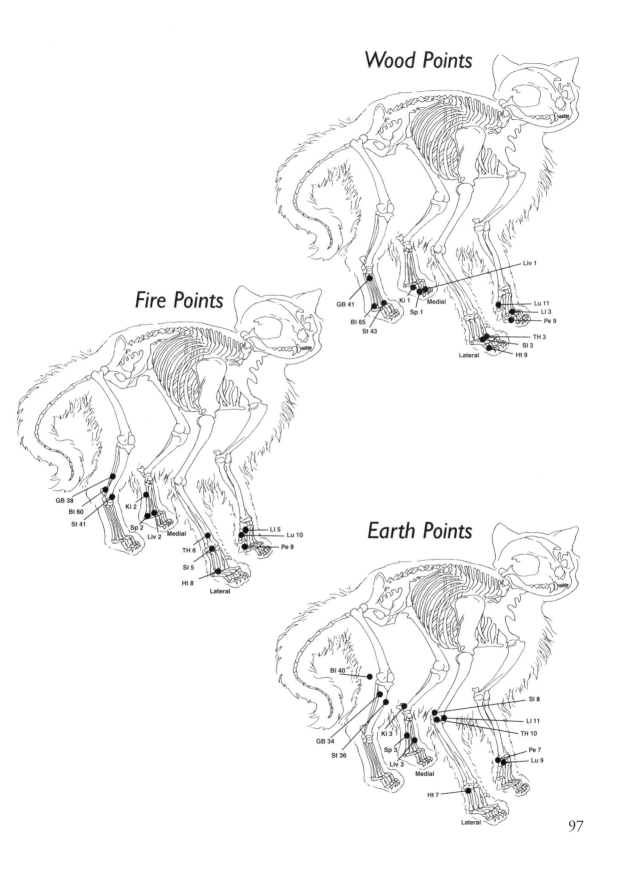

Wood Points

Liv 1
GB 41
Ki 1
Medial
Sp 1
Lu 11
LI 3
Pe 9
Bl 65
St 43
TH 3
Si 3
Lateral
Ht 9

Fire Points

GB 38
Bl 60
St 41
Ki 2
Sp 2
Liv 2
Medial
LI 5
Lu 10
Pe 8
TH 6
Si 5
Ht 8
Lateral

Earth Points

Bl 40
Si 8
LI 11
TH 10
GB 34
Ki 3
St 36
Sp 3
Liv 3
Medial
Pe 7
Lu 9
Ht 7
Lateral

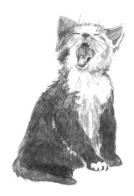

CONNECTING POINTS

Definition

The Connecting Points, also known as "luo" points, connect the Yin and Yang energies of sister meridians. Stimulation of these points balances the Chi between paired meridians. Therefore, an imbalance of energy between the sister meridians may be resolved by using these points.

Benefits

Eastern literature on the subject says, the Connecting Point of the sister meridians behave as somewhat of a "shortcircuit," allowing for the excess of energy to pass through the point from one sister meridian to the other. For instance, if there is a disharmony in the Lung meridian we can help balance it by stimulating the Large Intestine Connecting Point. The Connecting Points of a sister meridian are used in conjunction with the Source Point of the affected meridian. As an example: A cat with weak or deficient lungs may need the Lung Source Point (Lu 9) tonified. To enhance the Source Point's effect, the Connecting Point of the lung's associated meridian, the Large Intestine (LI 6) may be stimulated.

Location

The Connecting Points are located on the fore and hind legs of the cat. See the chart on the opposite page for specific locations.

Connecting Points

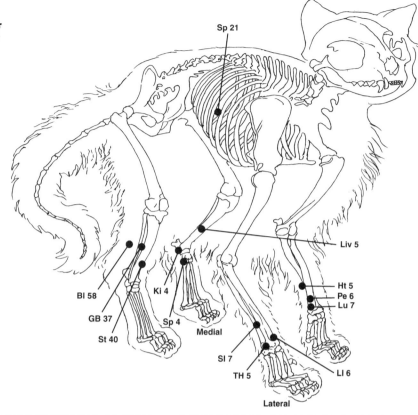

POINT	*TRADITIONAL NAME*	MERIDIAN OF CONNECTION
Lu 7	*Broken Sequence*	Large Intestine
LI 6	*Slanting Passage*	Lung
St 40	*Abundant Bulge*	Spleen
Sp 4	*Connecting Channels*	Stomach
Ht 5	*Inner Communication*	Small Intestine
SI 7	*Branch to Heart*	Heart
Bl 58	*Flying Up*	Kidney
Ki 4	*Big Bell*	Bladder
Pe 6	*Inner Gate*	Triple Heater
TH 5	*Outer Gate*	Pericardium
GB 37	*Brightness*	Liver
Liv 5	*Gourd Ditch*	Gall Bladder
Sp 21	*General Control*	Connecting Point for all Connecting Points

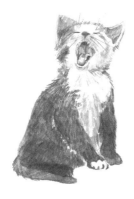

INFLUENTIAL POINTS

Definition

Influential Points can have a powerful affect on an entire functional system such as bones or tendons. These points are indicated for use in an ailment or problem associated with each point's sphere of influence or benefit.

Benefits

The Influential Points are highly effective and are commonly used in conjunction with other points to positively impact the treatment. For instance, in an older animal with a long-standing arthritic condition that has led to bone deformity, use the following point combination:

Bl 11   Influential Point for the bones
GB 39   Influential Point for marrow
St 40   Influential Point for phlegm
               (Spleen deficiency causing an accumulation of body fluids)

You may supplement these points with local points in the most affected areas. If the neck or head were involved, you can also add Lu 7, as the Master Point of that area.

Location

See chart on opposite page for specific location of the Influential Points.

Influential Points

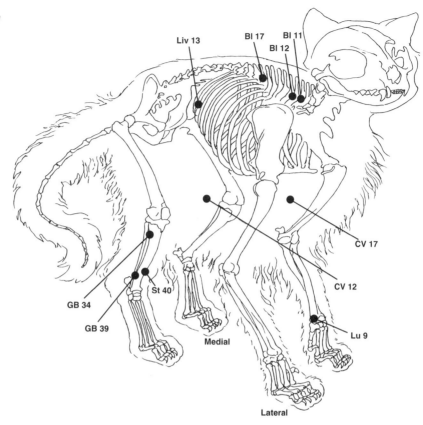

POINTS	*TRADITIONAL NAME*	AREA OF INFLUENCE
Lu 9	*Greater Abyss*	Arteries
Bl 11	*Big Reed*	Bones
Bl 12	*Wind Door*	Wind and trachea
Bl 17	*Back Transporting Point*	Blood and diaphragm
		Builds the immune system
St 40	*Abundant Bulge*	Phlegm
GB 34	*Yang Hill Spring*	Tendons
GB 39	*Hanging Bell*	Marrow and brain
Liv 13	*Chapter Gate*	Yin organs
CV 12	*Middle Epigastrium*	Yang organs
CV 17	*Middle of Chest*	Respiratory system and Chi

Note: Conception Vessel points are located on the ventral midline.

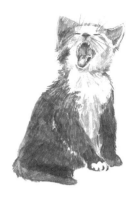

Master points

Definition

The Master Points powerfully affect a specific anatomical region of your cat's body such as the head and neck, or the back and hips. These points may be used for problems or ailments within the region of influence for each point. For example, you may want to use Bl 40, the Master Point for the back and hips, if your cat has back or hip trauma.

Benefits

By including a Master Point that affects a specific area of the body where there is an illness or injury, you can significantly enhance an acupressure treatment.

Location

The Master Points are located on the fore and hind legs, not necessarily in the area they impact. See chart on opposite page for specific location.

Master Points

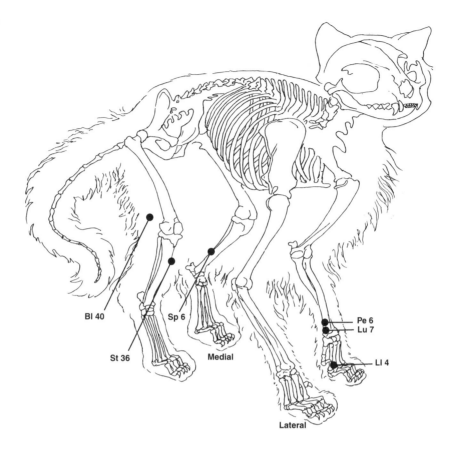

Bl 40 Sp 6 Pe 6 Lu 7 St 36 Medial LI 4 Lateral

POINTS	TRADITIONAL NAME	REGION OF IMPACT
LI 4	*Joining Valley*	Face and mouth
Lu 7	*Broken Sequence*	Head and neck
St 36	*Foot Three Miles*	Abdomen and gastrointestinal tract
Sp 6	*Three Yin Meeting*	Urogenital systems and the rear portion of the abdomen
Bl 40	*Supporting Middle*	Lower back and hips
Pe 6	*Inner Gate*	Chest and front portion of the abdomen

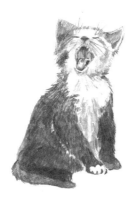

SEDATION POINTS

Definition

All twelve major meridians have a Sedation Point. A Sedation Point can subdue or disperse excess energy within the meridian flow. Sedation Points are often warm to the touch and protrude slightly from the body of the cat.

Benefits

Sedation Points are used to disperse or decrease energy in a meridian. For example, in a cat who angers easily, you may want to disperse the energy in the liver. To sedate the energy, work Liv 2, the Sedation Point on the Liver Meridian.

Location

The Sedation Points are located on the fore or hind legs of the cat along the organ meridian whose activity it governs. See the chart on the opposite page for specific location.

Sedation
Points

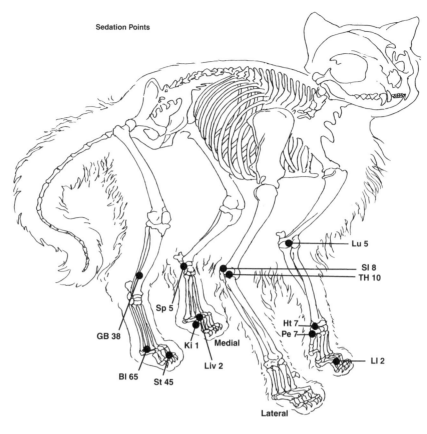

POINTS	*TRADITIONAL NAME*	MERIDIAN
Lu 5	*Foot Marsh*	Lung
LI 2	*Second Interval*	Large Intestine
St 45	*Sick Mouth*	Stomach
Sp 5	*Gold Mound*	Spleen
Ht 7	*Mind Door*	Heart
SI 8	*Small Intestine Sea*	Small Intestine
Bl 65	*Binding Bone*	Bladder
Ki 1	*Bubbling Spring*	Kidney
Pe 7	*Great Hill*	Pericardium
TH 10	*Heavenly Well*	Triple Heater
GB 38	*Yang Aid*	Gall Bladder
Liv 2	*Temporary In-Between*	Liver

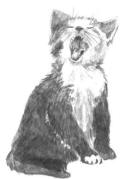

SOURCE POINTS

Definition

All twelve major meridians have a Source Point. They are identified by the organ on which they are located. The Source Point is located along the organ's meridian and can sedate or tonify depending on the specific need of the meridian at the time of the acupressure treatment. Swelling or deep dip at a point location indicates the need for Source Point work.

> Source Points are neutral, self-regulating and stabilizing. Although each point can be stimulated individually, it is more common to combine the Source Points of two or more organ systems during a treatment. For example, the sister meridian Source Points of Ki 3 and Bl 64 are used for urinary problems.

Benefit

Source Points can be used to determine if there is an excess or deficiency in an organ as well as restore the balance of Chi energy in their associated meridian. Source Point work can produce an immediate effect. In combination with a Tonification, Sedation or Association Point, the effect of either point work can be enhanced. Source points can also be used singularly or in combination with other points to help balance emotional or behavioral issues.

Source Points are particularly effective in tonifying the Yin organs. If your cat tends to have respiratory problems, in addition to the traditional treatment by your veterinarian, stimulation of the Lung Source Point can help to strengthen the Lung Meridian.

Location

The Source Points are located primarily around the wrist and hock of your cat. See the chart on the opposite page for their specific location.

Source Points

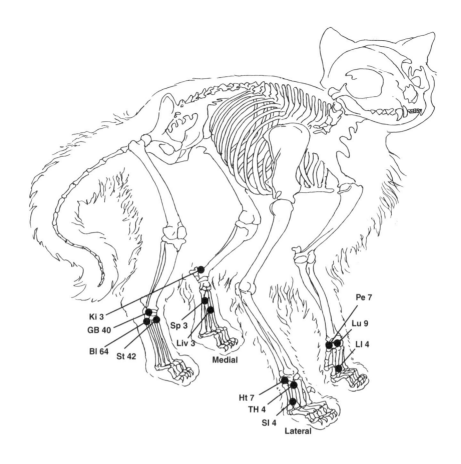

POINTS	TRADITIONAL NAME	MERIDIAN
Lu 9	*Greater Abyss*	Lung
LI 4	*Joining Valley*	Large Intestine
St 42	*Rushing Yang*	Stomach
Sp 3	*Greater White*	Spleen
Ht 7	*Mind Door*	Heart
SI 4	*Wrist Bone*	Small Intestine
Bl 64	*Capital Bone*	Bladder
Ki 3	*Greater Stream*	Kidney
Pe 7	*Great Hill*	Pericardium
TH 4	*Yang Pond*	Triple Heater
GB 40	*Mound Ruins*	Gall Bladder
Liv 3	*Bigger Rushing*	Liver

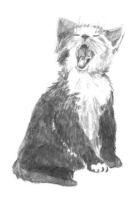

Ting points

Definition

Each of the twelve major meridians has a Ting Point. It is important to view the Ting Points in relation to each other. Unbalanced Ting Points may look and feel different from the other Ting Points and surrounding skin. This may indicate that there is an imbalance in the Ting Point's corresponding meridian. If a point feels warm, slightly swollen or protrudes, it may be an excess condition and possibly an acute situation. If a Ting Point feels soft and dips or a pit is left after pressure is released, and other characteristics like dry hair or skin are present, there is most likely a deficiency condition indicating a chronic situation.

Benefit

Ting Points provide important information regarding the general health and well-being of your cat. It is possible to detect meridian imbalances and disease by being aware of particular visual and tactile cues that Ting Points exhibit. They are very powerful points for treatment. There are practitioners who balance the whole cat by using Ting Points alone.

Location

Ting Points are located on the front and hind legs of the cat. Each Ting Point is either the beginning or end point of the meridian it impacts most directly. See the chart on the opposite page for the specific location of each Ting Point.

Ting Points

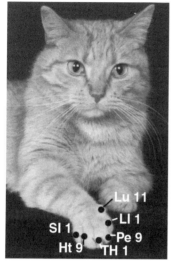

FORELEG

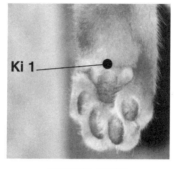

HIND LEG

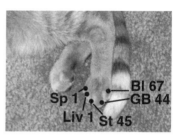

HIND LEG

POINTS	*TRADITIONAL NAME*	MERIDIAN
Lu 11	*Lesser Metal*	Lung
LI 1	*Metal Yang*	Large Intestine
St 45	*Sick Mouth*	Stomach
Sp 1	*Hidden White*	Spleen
Ht 9	*Lesser Yin Rushing*	Heart
SI 1	*Lesser Marsh*	Small Intestine
Bl 67	*Reaching Yin*	Bladder
Ki 1	*Bubbling Spring*	Kidney
Pe 9	*Center Rush*	Pericardium
TH 1	*Gate Rush*	Triple Heater
GB 44	*Orifice Yin*	Gall Bladder
Liv 1	*Big Thick*	Liver

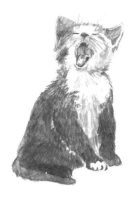

Tonification points

Definition

Each of the twelve major meridians has its own Tonification Point. These points are located on the meridian for which they are named. Stimulation of a Tonification Point will increase Chi energy in that meridian. These points usually feel cool to the touch.

Benefit

By working the Tonification Point you can increase Chi energy to the entire meridian and its corresponding organ. If your cat's Heart Meridian feels as if it is depleted, stimulation of the Tonification Point on the Heart Meridian, Ht 9, can add Chi energy to the Heart Meridian pathway.

Location

The Tonification Points are located on the fore and hind legs of your cat. See the chart on the opposite page for specific location.

Tonification Points

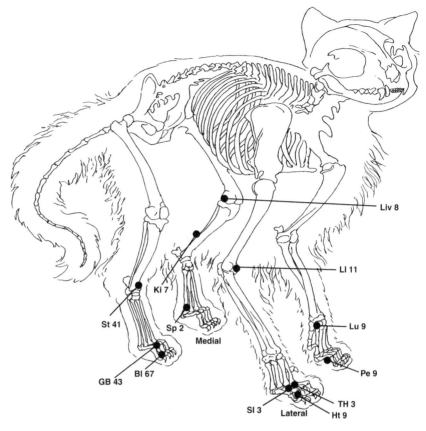

POINTS	TRADITIONAL NAME	MERIDIAN
Lu 9	*Greater Abyss*	Lung
LI 11	*Crooked Pond*	Large Intestine
St 41	*Dispersing Stream*	Stomach
Sp 2	*Big Capital*	Spleen
Ht 9	*Lesser Yin Rushing*	Heart
SI 3	*Back Stream*	Small Intestine
Bl 67	*Reaching Yin*	Bladder
Ki 7	*Returning Current*	Kidney
Pe 9	*Center Rush*	Pericardium
TH 3	*Middle Islet*	Triple Heater
GB 43	*Stream Insertion*	Gall Bladder
Liv 8	*Spring and Bend*	Liver

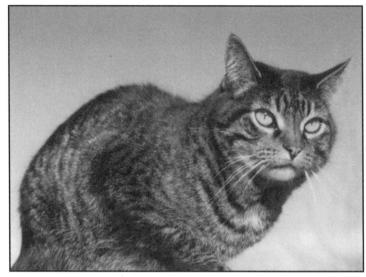

George

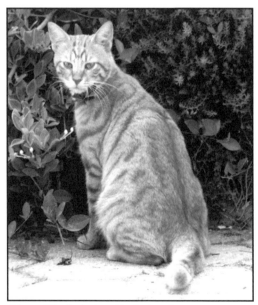

Photo: Elisabeth Apt, Haifa, Israel

Cats do not wear their hearts on their sleeves, which is not to say that they do not miss you when you are away. However, they feel that you have behaved very badly, and may not be civil when you return. After you have apologized, normal relations can be resumed.
—Susanne Millen

chapter six
Acupressure Treatments for Specific Conditions

From the minute Traditional Chinese Medicine practitioners meet their clients, they carefully observe the entire "aspect" of the person or cat. They are looking for signs of disharmony. The process of discerning imbalances, using the Four Examinations method, is extensive. It begins with a detailed physical observation in which the practitioner listens, smells, and touches the client. This is followed by asking in-depth questions about the client's nature, lifestyle, environment, and current complaint. During the examination process, TCM practitioners sort the information gathered into categories that lead to understanding distinguishing patterns.

In Chapter Two, Traditional Chinese Medicine, we briefly described the concepts underlying TCM. The Four Questions, the Eight Guiding Principles, the Six Layers, and the Five Phases of Transformation give you an idea of how thoroughly TCM practitioners are striving to understand the client's physical and psychological condition. It takes many years of study and practice to become truly competent in providing a holistic approach toward healthcare delivery. This manual can launch a journey toward learning acupressure and provide guidance in bringing some relief from common problems. When you are faced with a situation where your cat is ill or injured, we expect you to consult your holistic veterinarian and other animal healthcare providers to resolve a specific health issue.

TCM focuses on the natural transformation and balance of all things. All that exists must be in harmonious flow with itself and the universe from its beginnings to its ending. It is a never-ending cycle of birth, growth, maturity, harvesting the bounty of life and then passing. Cats have an inner sense and acceptance of the phases of their life-cycles. Perhaps this is what makes them seem so wise and pensive as they get on in years.

Kittens begin their tender lives with a lot of soft, fuzzy promise. Their eyes are sealed shut, their ears flattened against their heads and their shaky, fragile little bodies instinctively seek their mother for nourishment and warmth. From the moment of birth, cats have their own temperaments and individual needs. They are born with all the Source Chi they will ever have for the rest of their lives. Some are blessed with more and some with less.

Source Chi is the essence, or Jing, of life force energy and is the basis of all Yin and Yang energy in your cat's body throughout his life. If your kitten's queen and male live healthy, hardy lives and come from a line of well-cared-for cats, he will most likely start out with a full complement of Jing. Source Chi dissipates with age.

Since Source Chi cannot be replenished, it is up to you to help your cat preserve Jing by providing a healthy lifestyle. Cats require nourishing, protein-rich food, consistent physical exercise, and activities that challenge their keen hunting instincts. A balanced, active lifestyle also builds your cat's vital and replenishable spirit Chi, or Shen. Cats love to stalk bugs in grass or race down the hall after a furry mouse-like toy. Energizing activities in natural environments, fresh air, sunlight, and moonlight go a long way to building Shen and preserving Jing Chi.

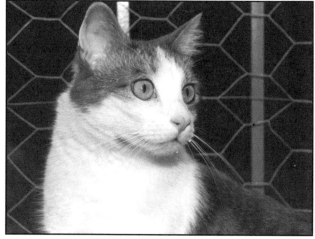

Energetic 3-year-old Baxter Cohen

Acupressure treatments in conjunction with other healing modalities contribute to the energetic life force every cat needs, but these must be accompanied by a good diet, physical exercise, a healthy environment and sensory stimulation to have good health and a long life.

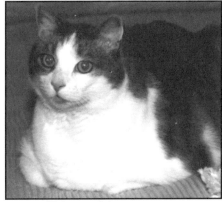

Baxter began life as an energetic, high-spirited, healthy fellow. His caregiver loved his bright amber-green eyes, gray and white face, slender, strong body, and affectionate nature. Baxter's guardian lavished hours of attention, bought the high-priced processed food, gave him everything she thought an apartment cat could want. Years passed and Baxter became lethargic. His body transformed into an unhealthy looking rotund

9-year-old Baxter Cohen

shape. His human had all good intentions, but Baxter became a "couch potato." She bought him processed low-fat diet food and kept reducing the amount of food she gave him in an effort to reduce his consistently expanding girth.

Many factors over six years contributed to Baxter's growing discomfort and potential for heart failure. His world was a small apartment with little opportunity for strenuous exercise. He was not deriving the appropriate nutrients from his food. He had little psychological stimulation to enliven his senses. Food, although it was not nourishing for him, had become Baxter's main source of pleasure and satisfaction. He meowed for more and ate it with relish when his caregiver indulged him.

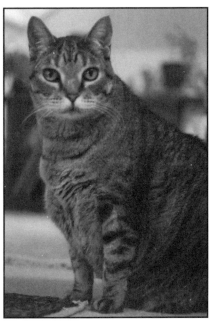

Obesity is one of the greatest problems we have in the domesticated cat population. For lack of other stimulation cats become obsessed with packaged food. Without the exercise that outdoor hunting expeditions gives them or an indoor substitute, cats will get fat. In Baxter's case, we used acupressure to address his lower back soreness caused by extra weight. We also suggested an Immune System Strengthening Treatment for his general health. Baxter's caregiver worked with a holistic veterinarian to increase the protein level

Sophie Soderberg

and quality of his food so that he could absorb more nutrients. She also bought him new indoor toys and activities and takes him for walks at a park nearby. Today, Baxter is eleven years old and enjoying the harvest years of his life as a slim, energetic, affectionate feline.

Specific Conditions

After an exhaustive examination in which the TCM practitioner determines the distinguishing pattern causing your cats' imbalance, he or she can arrive at a holistic course of action. Usually, the recommendation includes a combination of healing modalities to be used simultaneously. These healing arts include herbal remedies, exercise, meditation, dietary remedies, acupressure/ acupuncture, massage and other forms of body manipulation.

This chapter contains acupressure Point Work for more than 30 common feline physical and psychological complaints. The Point Work we recommend has shown to benefit many cats and other animals with similar ailments. When performing a treatment, begin with the standard Opening procedure described in Chapter Three, Feline Acupressure Treatment, then perform the Point Work provided in this chapter. Follow Point Work with

Acupoints

An acupoint can serve many purposes, depending on the body's condition. Don't be surprised to find that a point is known for its calming effects, while it also relieves chronic tiredness, reduces pain and regulates the uterus and estrous cycle (Spleen 6, Three Yin Meeting).

Large Intestine 4, Joining Valley, has several healing attributes. It is listed in many treatment plans: Immune Strengthening, Shoulder Soreness, Pain Reduction, Arthritis, Constipation, Skin Conditions, and Vision Treatments. Rather than list all the attributes under each condition, only the applicable attributes are listed for specific conditions.

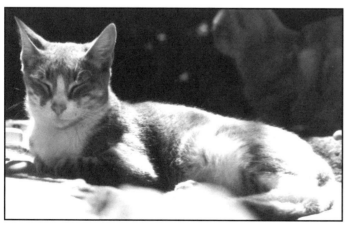

the Closing procedure. Conditions such as trauma or shock require immediate attention from your veterinarian. You can perform the acupressure treatment suggested in this chapter while your cat is in transit to the veterinary clinic. Acupressure is a complement to veterinary medicine, not a substitute.

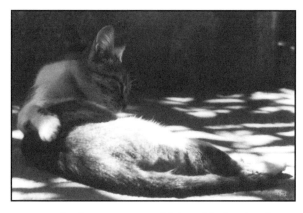

Because each cat differs from all others, you may find that your cat improves significantly after using only some of the points listed for the condition. Feel free to adapt the recommended Point Work to your cat's particular needs. After he has experienced a few treatments, he most likely will show you which points need attention, by scratching or licking a particular spot or rubbing his body along a meridian.

There are two essential elements in acupressure work. The first is to trust your cat's and your own sense of healing. The second is to provide treatments consistently. When trust in your healing abilities combines with ongoing treatment, the results are powerful.

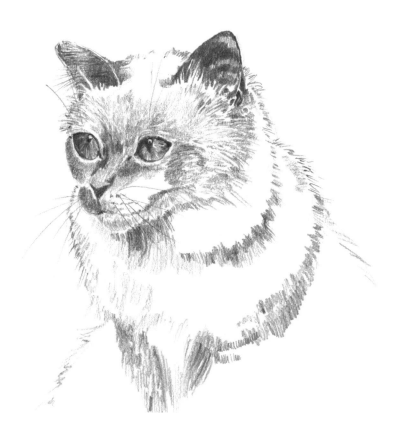

Arthritis

In recent years we have seen an increase in arthritic conditions in cats. TCM has demonstrated its capacity to relieve many arthritic conditions. Selection of a treatment plan depends on where the arthritis is located and when the condition appears. After observing when and where your cat's arthritis is exhibited, select the appropriate treatment.

Indicators

Specific joint soreness or inflammation
Stiff or impeded movement of joints
Difficulty with stairs

Heat around the joints
Difficulty jumping

WORSE WITH COLD

Presentation of Arthritis

Worse with Cold
Arthritic area may feel cold, joints as well as muscles may be involved.

Procedure
Open the Stomach, Large Intestine and Conception Vessel Meridians along their entire length on both sides of your cat.

Perform specific Point Work on **St 36, LI 10 and 11 & CV 6**

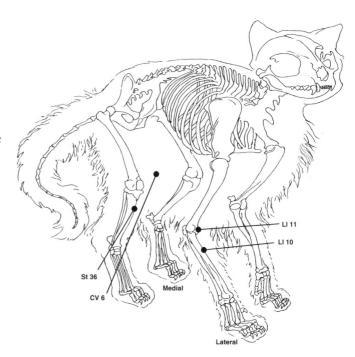

POINT	*TRADITIONAL NAME*	FUNCTION
St 36	*Leg Three Miles*	Benefits the immune system. Tonifies Chi and blood and regulates the circulation of Chi. Best point to work to improve strength, health and resistance to disease.
LI 10	*Hand Three Miles*	Relieves arthritic conditions.
LI 11	*Pond on the Curve*	Tonification Point. Benefits the immune system, use for arthritic conditions particularly of the elbow and foreleg.
CV 6	*Sea of Chi*	Benefits Chi as a general tonifying effect.

Note: Conception Vessel points are located on the ventral midline of your cat.

JOINTS EXHIBIT HEAT

Presentation of Arthritis

Joints Exhibit Heat   Arthritis presents suddenly, joints are swollen and painful. Pain increases with pressure.

Procedure   Open the Large Intestine, Stomach and Governing Vessel Meridians along their entire length on both sides of your cat. Perform specific on **LI 4 and 11, St 44 and GV 14**

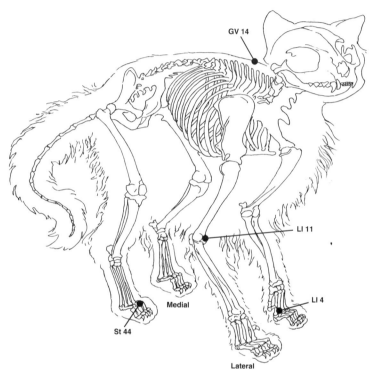

POINT	*TRADITIONAL NAME*	FUNCTION
LI 4	*Joining Valley*	Source Point. Relieves pain in any part of the body.
LI 11	*Pond on the Curve*	Tonification Point. Benefits the immune system, use for arthritic conditions particularly of the elbow and foreleg.
St 44	*Inner Courtyard*	Use for arthritic conditions, clears heat.
GV 14	*Big Vertebra*	Meeting point of all Yang meridians. Strengthens the immune system and clears heat.

WORSE IN WET WEATHER
Presentation of Arthritis

Worse in Wet Weather	Condition presents more stiff than painful. Edema around joint and down the leg. Living in a damp environment can cause this condition.
Procedure	Open the Stomach, Spleen and Conception Vessel Meridians along their entire length on both sides of your cat. Perform specific at **St 36 & 40, Sp 6 & 9, and CV 4**

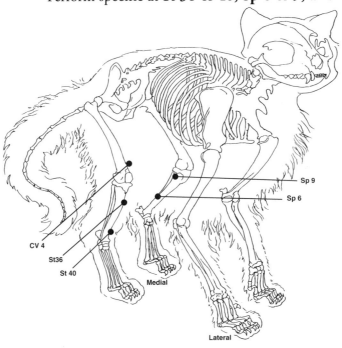

POINT	*TRADITIONAL NAME*	FUNCTION
St 36	*Leg Three Miles*	Tonification Point. Benefits the immune system and regulates the circulation of Chi.
St 40	*Abundant Bulge*	Connecting Point. Reduces hind limb swelling and clears dampness.
Sp 6	*Three Yin Meeting*	Junction of three Yin channels: Spleen, Kidney and Liver. Benefits the immune system. Do not stimulate this point during pregnancy.
Sp 9	*Yin Mound Spring*	Benefits the Spleen. Main point for reducing dampness.
CV 4	*Gate to the Original*	Benefits the Kidneys and Yin. Strengthens the general energy level.

Note: Conception Vessel points are located on the ventral midline of your cat.

120

LOCATION OF PAIN CHANGES

Presentation of Arthritis
Location of Pain Changes

Arthritic pain moves around the body. Muscles as well as joints are sore. May be worse during or after windy weather.

Procedure

Perform specific at **LI 11, Bl 11 & 12, TH 5, GB 39, and GV 14**

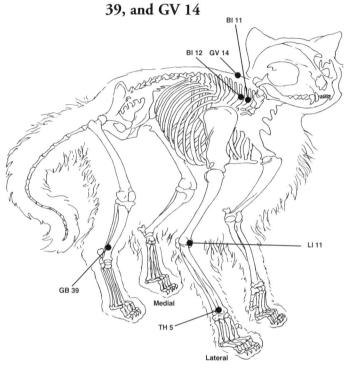

POINT	*TRADITIONAL NAME*	FUNCTION
LI 11	*Pond on the Curve*	Tonification Point. Benefits the immune system.
Bl 11	*Big Reed*	Influential Point for bone. Helps relieve arthritic pain. Tonifies the blood and Protective and Nutritive Chi.
Bl 12	*Wind Door*	Relieves cervical pain. Disperses Chi.
TH 5	*Outer Gate*	Reduces arthritic pain especially of the wrist, elbow and shoulder.
GB 39	*Hanging Bell*	Influential Point for bone marrow. Strengthens the immune system.
GV 14	*Big Vertebra*	Master Point for all Yang meridians. Strengthens the immune system.

Ear Problems

HEARING LOSS

Indicators

Not responding to loud
stimuli
General reduction of
activity
Reluctance or refusal to
go outside
Startled responses

Procedure

Open the Small
Intestine, Triple Heater
and Gall Bladder
Meridians. Perform specific
Point Work on **SI 19,
TH 5 & 21 and GB 2**

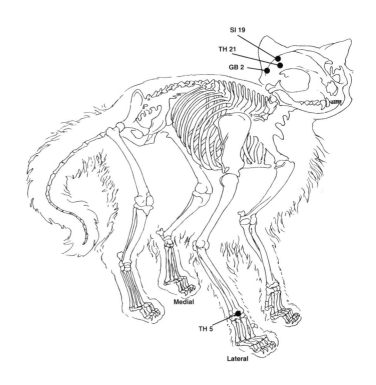

POINT	TRADITIONAL NAME	FUNCTION
SI 19	Listening Palace	Benefits the ears. Meeting place of Small Intestine, Gall Bladder and Triple Burner.
TH 5	Outer Gate	Benefits the ear, use for ear infections or hearing deficiency.
TH 21	Ear Door	Use as local point for ear problems and diminished hearing.
GB 2	Hearing Convergence	Important local point for ear problems and diminished hearing.

122

EAR INFECTION/ACHE

Indicators

Excessive head shaking

Ear discharge or odor

Redness around the ear

Pain when touched around the ear

Procedure

Open the Small Intestine, Triple Heater and Large Intestine Meridians.
Perform specific Point Work on **SI 19, TH 5, 7 & 17 and LI 4 & 11**

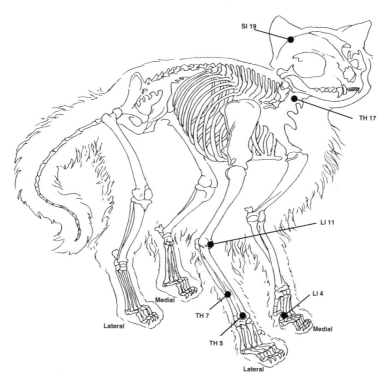

POINT	*TRADITIONAL NAME*	FUNCTION
SI 19	*Listening Palace*	Benefits the ears. Meeting place of Small Intestine, Gall Bladder and Triple Heater.
TH 5	*Outer Gate*	Benefits the ear, use for ear infections or hearing deficiency.
TH 7	*Converging Channels*	Benefits the ears and eyes. Stops pain.
TH 17	*Wind Screen*	Benefits the ears.
LI 4	*Joining Valley*	Relieves pain. Has a strong influence on the face. Positive affect on infection.
LI 11	*Pond on the Curve*	Builds the immune system.

Eye Problems

EYE INFLAMMATION

Indicators

Red or swollen eyes
Yellow discharge from eyes
Excessive tearing
Crusty discharge and
difficulty opening eyes

Procedure

Open the Bladder, Large
Intestine, Gall Bladder and
Governing Vessel Meridians.
Perform specific Point Work
on **BL 1, 2 & 67,
LI 4 & 11, GB 37
and GV 14**

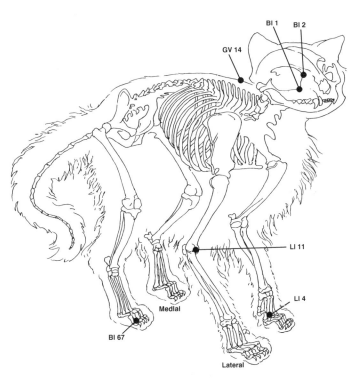

POINT	TRADITIONAL NAME	FUNCTION
Bl 1	Eye Brightness	Powerful point for all eye problems.
Bl 2	Collecting Bamboo	Brightens the eye, calms the Liver and stops pain.
Bl 67	Reaching Yin	Use to clear the eyes and invigorate blood.
LI 4	Joining Valley	Relieves pain. Has a strong influence on the face. Positive affect on infection.
LI 11	Pond on the Curve	Builds the immune system.
GB 37	Brightness	Use for all eye disorders. Improves sight.
GV 14	Big Vertebra	Strengthens the immune system.

VISION PROBLEMS

Indicators

Onset of cataracts

Lack of awareness of moving objects

Walking or running into objects

Fear of going outside

Consistent defensive behavior

Procedure

Open the Bladder, Stomach and Gall Bladder Meridians.

Perform specific Point Work on **Bl 1 & 67, St 1& 8 and GB 20 & 37**

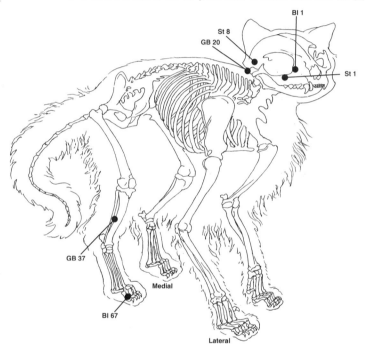

POINT	TRADITIONAL NAME	FUNCTION
Bl 1	*Eye Brightness*	Benefits eye disorders of both internal and external origin. Use for all eye disorders.
Bl 67	*Reaching Yin*	Tonification Point. Clears the eyes of blurred vision or pain.
St 1	*Containing Tears*	Used for eye problems including, conjunctivitis, cataract and glaucoma.
St 8	*Head Support*	Benefits and brightens the eyes, relieves pain.
GB 20	*Wind Pond*	Benefits the eyes Helps blurred vision and cataracts.
GB 37	*Brightness*	Improves eyesight and removes floaters in the eyes. Use to treat all eye disorders.

125

Gastrointestinal Disorders

Consult your veterinarian if your cat experiences diarrhea or constipation for even a short period of time. Diarrhea can cause dehydration very quickly. Constipation can be caused by unsuitable diet or a bowel obstruction. Constipation is a common problem in older cats.

CONSTIPATION

Indicators

Difficult, infrequent or
absent bowel movement
Loss of appetite, vomiting,
dehydration or a hunched
back due to a tummy ache

Procedure

Open the Large Intestine,
Bladder, Stomach, Spleen
and Triple Heater
Meridians along their
entire length on both
sides of your cat. Perform
specific Point Work on
**LI 2, Bl 25, St 36,
Sp 6 and TH 6**

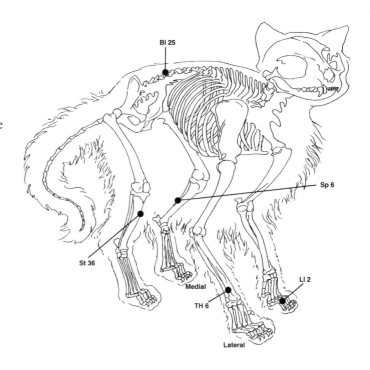

POINT	*TRADITIONAL NAME*	FUNCTION
LI 2	*Second Interval*	Relieves constipation by clearing heat.
Bl 25	*Large Intestine Transporting Point*	Promotes excreting function of the large intestine, relieves abdominal fullness and distension.
St 36	*Leg Three Miles*	Benefits the stomach and spleen.
Sp 6	*Three Yin Meeting*	Master Point for lower abdomen.
TH 6	*Branching Ditch*	Removes obstructions from the large intestine.

DIARRHEA

Indicators

Soft or loose stools
Abundant stools
Mucous in stools

Procedure

Open the Large Intestine, Bladder, Stomach, and Spleen Meridians along their entire length on both sides of your cat.
Perform specific Point Work on **LI 4, Bl 20, St 25 & 36, and Sp 6 & 9**

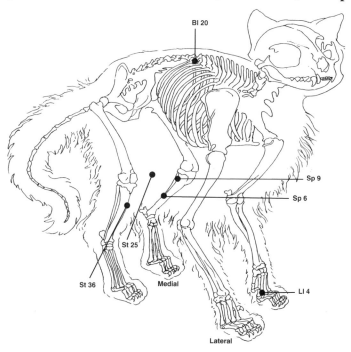

POINT	TRADITIONAL NAME	FUNCTION
LI 4	*Joining Valley*	Balances the gastrointestinal system.
Bl 20	*Spleen Back Transporting Point*	Calms digestive disorders.
St 25	*Heavenly Pillar*	Use for gastrointestinal disorders, relieves diarrhea.
St 36	*Leg Three Miles*	Benefits and strengthens stomach and spleen.
Sp 6	*Three Yin Meeting*	Master Point for lower abdomen. Strengthens the spleen and resolves damp heat.
Sp 9	*Yin Mound Spring*	Relieves diarrhea.

INDIGESTION

Indicators

Unusually loud, long gut sounds
Unusual dispelling of gas

Vomiting
Suppressed appetite

Procedure

Open the Stomach, Pericardium and Conception Vessel Meridians along their entire length on both sides of your cat.
Perform specific Point Work on **St 25, 36 & 44, Pe 6 and CV 12 & 14**

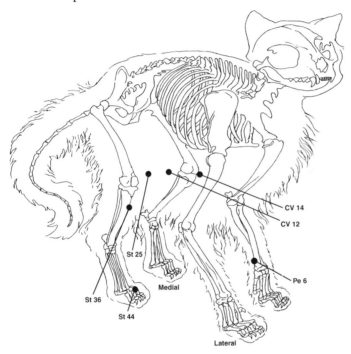

Cats efficiently expel toxic or harmful substances by vomiting. They clear their digestive system of hairballs and other irritants often. If your cat is vomiting frequently without an obvious cause, losing weight or refusing to eat, consult your veterinarian immediately.

POINT	TRADITIONAL NAME	FUNCTION
St 25	*Heavenly Pillar*	Relieves food retention and acute patterns of the stomach.
St 36	*Leg Three Miles*	Benefits the stomach and spleen.
St 44	*Inner Courtyard*	Promotes digestion and relieves pain.
Pe 6	*Inner Gate*	Calms indigestion and calms the spirit.
CV 12	*Middle of Epigastrium*	Regulates Stomach Chi, use for any digestive disorder.
CV 14	*Great Palace*	Relieves digestive disorders, especially from an emotional origin.

Note: Conception Vessel points are located on the ventral midline of your cat.

GUM PROBLEMS

Indicators

Red or swollen gums   Weight loss
Spongy, ulcerated or bleeding gums
Unusually bad breath
Chewing on one side of mouth

Procedure

Open the Bladder, Liver, Large Intestine, Stomach and
Conception Vessel Meridians.
Perform specific Point Work at **Bl 20, Liv 3, LI 4,
St 44 and CV 12**

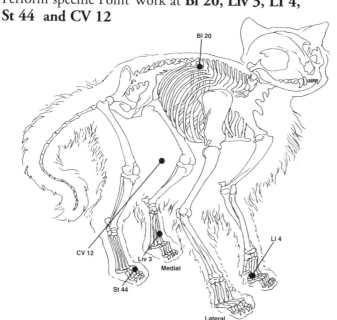

Natural Foods
    A cat's natural diet of rodents, birds and bugs not only provides the nutrients and roughage a cat needs but also the chewing, teeth cleaning and gum stimulation needed for oral and psychological health. When commercially processed food were introduced for ease of feeding pets, cats lost the benefits of their natural diet. We recommend giving your cat chicken or turkey bones to chew and slowly introducing some raw meats along with processed food.

POINT	TRADITIONAL NAME	FUNCTION
Bl 20	Spleen Back Transporting Point	Nourishes the blood. Reinforce this point for chronic conditions with depleted energy.
Liv 3	Bigger Rushing	Major point used to sedate Liver excess. Affects and calms the head.
LI 4	Joining Valley	Master Point for the face and head. Helps stop pain.
St 44	Inner Courtyard	Stops pain, clears heat and benefits weak, bleeding gums.
CV 12	Middle of Epigastrium	Relates to the Spleen energy center. On a physical level is responsible for digestion from mouth to intestines.

Note: Conception Vessel points are located on the ventral midline of your cat.

Hip Dysplasia

Until recently hip dysplasia was considered canine-specific. Unfortunately hip dysplasia has become prevalent in the general feline population. It is seen in small and large cats alike. Feline hip dysplasia (FHD) is a painful malformation of the hip joint which becomes apparent as the cat matures. Although diet is considered a contributing factor, some cats have an hereditary predisposition to developing hip dysplasia and other orthopedic conditions. The suggested Point Work for hip dysplasia addresses pain reduction, bone and joint issues, associated arthritis and strengthening of the immune system.

Indicators

Restricted hind limb mobility, lameness
Reluctance or inability to jump
Difficulty getting up or lying down
Hindquarter stiffness and sensitivity to touch

Procedure

Open the Bladder, Spleen, Gall Bladder and Liver Meridians along their entire length on both sides of your cat.
Perform specific Point Work on **Bl 11, 40 & 60, Sp 9, GB 29, 30 & 34 and Liv 3**

Note: Along with the acupressure treatment, an Animal Chiropractor is often helpful with resolving this condition

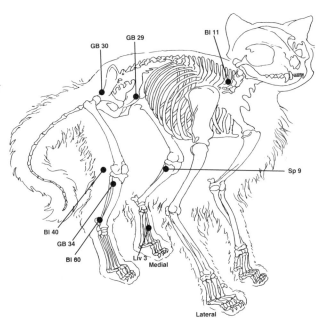

POINT	TRADITIONAL NAME	FUNCTION
Bl 11	*Big Reed*	Use for any bone or joint disorder, enhances bone healing and dispels wind.
Bl 40	*Entrusting Middle*	Master Point for lower back and hips. Use for arthritis in stifle, hip and back.
Bl 60	*Kunlun Mountain*	Aspirin Point. Use for arthritic conditions.
Sp 9	*Yin Mound Spring*	Use for pelvic problems, resolves dampness.
GB 29	*Squatting Crevice*	Use for disorders of joints, especially the hips.
GB 30	*Jumping Circle*	Use for hip soreness or dysplasia problems. Relaxes tendons and restores joint mobility.
GB 34	*Yang Spring Mound*	Relieves joint stiffness. Influential Point for the muscles and tendons.
Liv 3	*Bigger Rushing*	Relieves muscle spasms.

Immune System Strengthening

Indicators

Low-level infections
Presentation of allergic conditions
(eye or nasal discharge,
chronic skin problems)
Exposure to animals with
contagious conditions
Following a surgery, trauma
or a vaccination reaction

Procedure

Open the Large Intestine,
Bladder, Stomach, Spleen,
Conception and Governing
Vessel Meridians.
Perform Point Work on
**LI 4 & 11, Bl 18 & 23,
St 36, Sp 6, CV 6 and GV 14**

Frequency

Administer the acupressure
treatment every third day for
nine days or until the condition
is resolved.

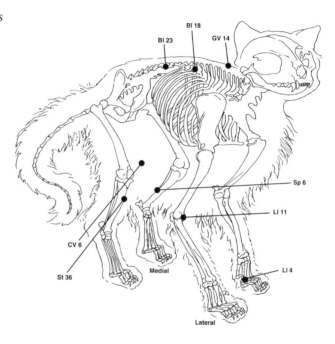

POINT	TRADITIONAL NAME	FUNCTION
LI 4	Joining Valley	Strengthens the immune system.
LI 11	Pond on the Curve	Relieves immune system weakness.
Bl 18	Liver Back Transporting Point	Supports the liver as a detoxifying agent.
Bl 23	Kidney Back Transporting	Strengthens the immune system. Nourishes Blood and Kidney essence. Supports detoxification of kidneys.
St 36	Leg Three Miles	Restores and strengthens the immune system. Generally improves strength, health and resistance to diseases.
Sp 6	Three Yin Meeting	Stimulates the body's immune system. Relieves chronic tiredness.
CV 6	Sea of Energy	Strengthens the immune system and internal organs. Represents the energy center of the body, stores and distributes energy.
GV 14	Big Vertebra	Strengthens the immune system.

Note: Conception Vessel points are located on the ventral midline of your cat.

Lower Back Soreness

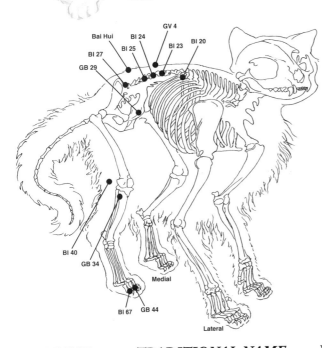

Bai Hui · BI 24 · GV 4 · BI 27 · BI 25 · BI 23 · BI 20 · GB 29

BI 40
GB 34
Medial
BI 67 · GB 44
Lateral

Indicators

Resistance to being touched or
groomed on the lower back
Difficulty jumping, climbing or
descending stairs
Uneven hind leg stride

Procedure

Open the Bladder, Gall Bladder
and Governing Vessel Meridians.
Perform specific Point Work on
**Bl 20, 23, 24, 25, 27, 40 & 67,
GB 29, 34 & 44, GV 4
and Bai Hui Point**

Frequency

Administer the acupressure treatment
every third day for nine days or
until the condition is resolved.

Note: Along with the acupressure
treatment, an Animal Chiropractor
is often helpful with resolving this
condition.

POINT	TRADITIONAL NAME	FUNCTION
Bl 20	Spleen Back Transporting Point	Relieves back pain and increases energy.
Bl 23	Kidney Back Transporting Point	Relieves chronic lower back and lumbosacral pain.
Bl 24	Sea of Chi Back Transporting Point	Relieves lumbosacral pain and moves stagnant Chi.
Bl 25	Lg Intestine Back Transporting Point	Relieves lower back pain.
Bl 27	Sm Intestine Back Transporting Point	Relieves sciatica and lower back pain.
Bl 40	Entrusting Middle	Master Point for the lower back. Relieves lumbar pain.
Bl 67	Reaching Yin	Ting Point. Benefits the lower back.
GB 29	Squatting Crevice	Relieves hindquarter muscle soreness and joint disorders.
GB 34	Yang Spring Mound	Strengthens the back and joints.
GB 44	Orifice Yin	Ting Point. Benefits the lower back.
GV 4	Gates of Life	Strengthens lower back, helps chronic back pain.
Bai Hui	Hundred Meetings	Relieves pain or lameness of the hindquarters. Use for pelvic limb or lumbar disorder.

Neutering and Spaying

As a responsible animal caretaker, you know that neutering your cat can add to the quality of his life. Consult with your holistic veterinarian for the best time to neuter and what other natural treatments, food or exercise are available to assist in his healing.

The points noted below will benefit your cat post surgery. These are general pain relief, muscle, soft tissue injury and immune system strengthening points. You can work these points every other day. Pay close attention to your animals comfort level when working this set of acupoints.

Procedure

Open the Large Intestine, Bladder, Stomach, and Spleen Meridians. Perform specific Point Work on **LI 11, Bl 60, St 36, Sp 6, 10 & 21**

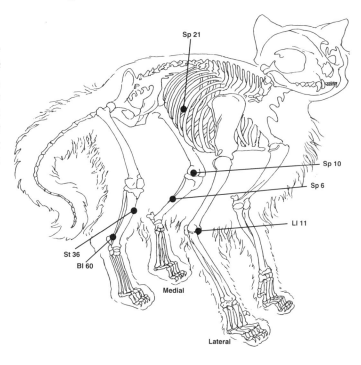

POINT	TRADITIONAL NAME	FUNCTION
LI 11	*Crooked Pond*	Tonification Point. Enhances immune system and relieves pain.
Bl 60	*Kunlun Mountains*	Reduces pain, clears heat and strengthens blood.
St 36	*Leg Three Miles*	Restores and strengthens the immune sytem. Generally improves strength, health and resistance to diseases.
Sp 6	*Three Yin Meeting*	Stops pain and moves blood, helps calm the mind.
Sp 10	*Sea of Blood*	Immune enhancing and blood tonifying point.
Sp 21	*General Control*	Reduces muscular pain throughout the body.

Respiratory Problems

The points chosen for Asthma, Bronchitis and Dry Cough are to be used in conjunction with holistic or traditional veterinary care. If your cat presents any of these conditions see your veterinarian immediately because breathing problems are life-threatening.

Asthma

Indicators
Recurring episodes of
  difficult breathing
Fatigues easily
Wheezing
Cough with mucous

Procedure
Open the Lung, Bladder, Stomach, Kidney and Conception Vessel Meridians. Perform Point Work on **Lu 5 & 7, Bl 20, St 12 & 40, Ki 27 and CV 17 & 22**

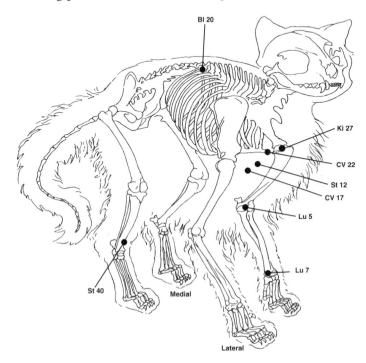

POINT	TRADITIONAL NAME	FUNCTION
Lu 5	Foot Marsh	Aids in respiratory conditions, dispels wind.
Lu 7	Broken Sequence	Use for acute or chronic cough or asthma conditions. Stimulates lung functions.
Bl 20	Spleen Back Transporting	Benefits the lungs.
St 12	Empty Basin	Calms Chi and relieves asthma.
St 40	Abundant Bulge	Clears asthma, heat and opens the chest. Resolves phlegm and damp.
Ki 27	Transporting Point Mansion	Local point for treating asthma.
CV 17	Middle of the Chest	Influential Point for the respiratory system. Clears the lungs, relieves fullness from the chest, tonifies Chi.
CV 22	Heaven Projection	Benefits acute and chronic cough and asthma.

Note: Conception Vessel points are located on the ventral midline of your cat.

Bronchitis

Indicators

Rough cough   Difficulty breathing

Lethargic attitude

Procedure

Open the Lung, Bladder, Pericardium, Governing and Conception Vessel Meridians.
Perform specific Point Work on **Lu 5, 8 & 9, Bl 12 & 13, Pe 6, GV 4 and CV 17**

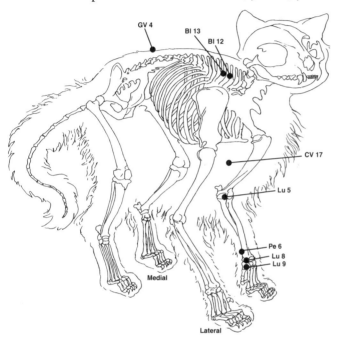

For cats with respiratory
problems be sure to avoid:
- Aerosol sprays
- Air fresheners
- Household cleaning
  chemicals
- Flea protection products
- Fertilizing chemicals
- Powdered carpet fresheners
- Smoke of any kind

POINT	TRADITIONAL NAME	FUNCTION
Lu 5	Foot Marsh	Aids in respiratory conditions, dispels wind.
Lu 8	Channel Canal	Use to treat conditions of throat and lungs.
Lu 9	Greater Abyss	Lung Source Point, transform phlegm.
Bl 12	Wind Door	Stimulates the functions of the lungs.
Bl 13	Lung Back Transporting Point	Strengthens Lung Chi, stimulates lungs.
Pe 6	Inner Gate	Master Point for chest & cranial abdomen.
GV 4	Gate of Life	Nourishes Original Chi, relieves tiredness and lack of vitality.
CV 17	Middle of the Chest	Influential Point for the respiratory system. Clears the lungs, relieves fullness from the chest, tonifies Chi.

Note: Conception Vessel points are located on the ventral midline of your cat.

DRY COUGH/LUNG CONGESTION

Indicators

Dry cough   Lethargic attitude

Procedure

Open the Lung and Conception Vessel Meridians.
Perform specific Point Work on **Lu 1, 5 & 7 and CV 22**

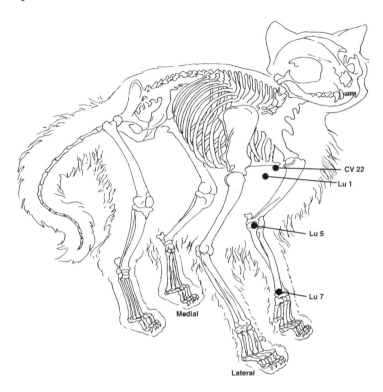

POINT	*TRADITIONAL NAME*	FUNCTION
Lu 1	*Central Residence*	Regulates Lung Chi and stops cough. Relieves pain.
Lu 5	*Foot Marsh*	Aids in respiratory conditions, dispels wind.
Lu 7	*Broken Sequence*	Opens the nose. Stimulates functions of the lungs and is an important point for acute or chronic coughs or asthma.
CV 22	*Heaven Projection*	Stimulates Lung Chi, use for acute and chronic coughs and asthma.

Note: Conception Vessel points are located on the ventral midline of your cat.

136

Shoulder Soreness

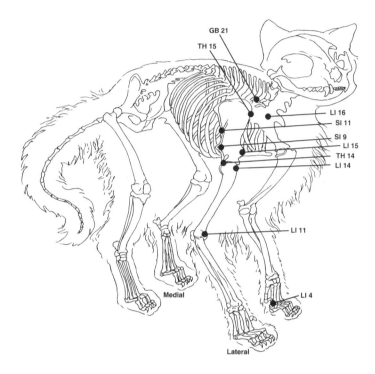

Indicators

Restricted forelimb mobility
Shuffling or uneven walk
Imbalanced development of
shoulder muscles

Procedure

Open the Large Intestine,
Small Intestine, Triple Heater
and Gall Bladder Meridians
along their entire length on both
sides of your cat.
Perform Point Work on
**LI 4, 11, 14 ,15 & 16,
SI 9 & 11, TH 14 &15
and GB 21**

Frequency

Administer treatment every third
day for twelve days or until
shoulder soreness is relieved.

Note: Along with the acupressure
treatment, an Animal Chiropractor is
often helpful with resolving this condition

POINT	*TRADITIONAL NAME*	FUNCTION
LI 4	*Joining Valley*	Relieves shoulder pain.
LI 11	*Crooked Pond*	Benefits joint, relieves pain in shoulder.
LI 14	*Upper Arm*	Relieves shoulder tension and relaxes shoulder muscles.
LI 15	*Shoulder Bone*	Relieves shoulder and elbow arthritis.
LI 16	*Great Bone*	Benefits joints, relieves shoulder pain.
SI 9	*Upright Shoulder*	Local point to relieve shoulder pain.
SI 11	*Heavenly Attribution*	Local point to relieve shoulder pain.
TH 14	*Shoulder Crevice*	Helps relieve shoulder pain.
TH 15	*Heavenly Crevice*	Local point for shoulder problems.
GB 21	*Shoulder Well*	Relieves shoulder pain and arthritis.

Skin Problems

In TCM terms, skin problems are seen as excessive heat conditions. The intent of a treatment plan is to reduce the inflammation while also strengthening the immune system. The following treatment plans include general points only and we suggest you consult your holistic veterinarian immediately. In response to anxiety or boredom, cats can obsessively lick or chew their own skin, causing sores. Environmental irritants, such as household cleaning chemicals, pesticides and fertilizers, are also known to cause skin inflammation and toxic reactions.

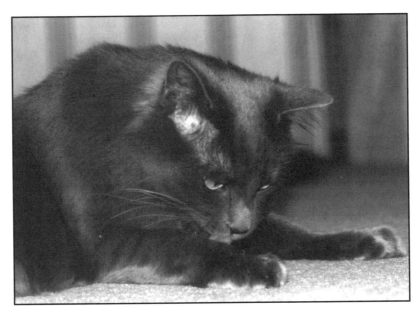

Fredd Jones

BLISTER OR RASH DISORDERS

Indicators

Excessive licking in one area   Crusty sores or scabs
Eruption of red, open sore   Loss of hair

Procedure

Open the Large Intestine, Bladder, Stomach Spleen & Governing Vessel Meridians.
Perform specific Point Work on **LI 11, Bl 11, 17, 23 & 40, St 44, Sp 9 and GV 14**

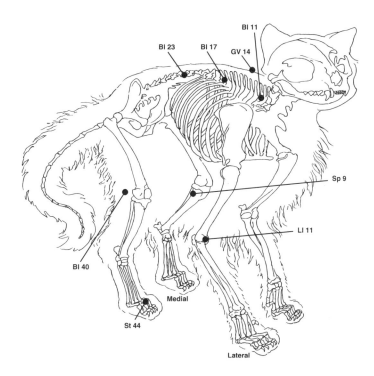

POINT	TRADITIONAL NAME	FUNCTION
LI 11	*Crooked Pond*	Enhances immune system.
Bl 11	*Big Reed*	Nourishes blood, strengthens Nutritive Chi, reduces pathogens.
Bl 17	*Diaphragm Back Transporting Point*	Benefits non-responsive skin conditions, relieves itchy skin.
Bl 23	*Kidney Back Transporting Point*	Stimulates the production of cortisone, anti-inflammatory.
Bl 40	*Supporting Middle*	Relieves skin conditions characterized by heat.
St 44	*Inner Courtyard*	Regulates the skin, reduces rashes or boils.
Sp 9	*Yin Mound Spring*	Relieves allergic and toxic conditions.
GV 14	*Big Vertebra*	Enhances immune system.

ITCHY, DRY SKIN

Indicators

Excessive scratching	Loss of hair
Excessive dander	Lackluster condition
Brittle and dry coat	

Procedure

Open the Lung, Large Intestine, Spleen, Triple Heater & Governing Vessel Meridians. Perform specific Point Work on **Lu 7, LI 4 & 11, Sp 6 & 9, TH 6 and GV 14**

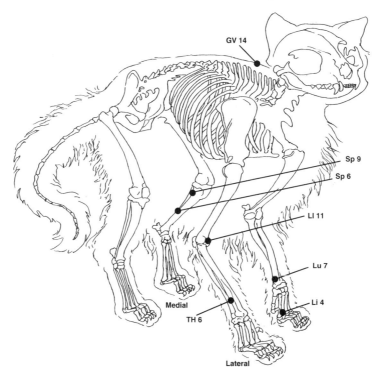

POINT	*TRADITIONAL NAME*	FUNCTION
Lu 7	*Broken Sequence*	Connecting Point. Strengthens lungs, benefits skin conditions.
LI 4	*Joining Valley*	Source Point. Enhances immune system.
LI 11	*Crooked Pond*	Enhances immune system.
Sp 6	*Three Yin Meeting*	Benefits skin conditions.
Sp 9	*Yin Mound Spring*	Relieves allergic and toxic conditions.
TH 6	*Branching Ditch*	Benefits itchy skin and skin diseases.
GV 14	*Big Vertebra*	Enhances immune system.

SKIN ALLERGIES

Indicators

Excessive scratching   Excessive licking of body
Eruption of sores   Change of body odor

Procedure

Open the Large Intestine, Bladder and Spleen Meridians along their entire length on both sides of your cat.

Perform specific Point Work on **LI 4 & 11, Bl 13 and Sp 6 & 9**

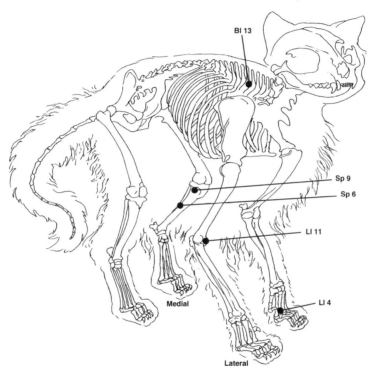

POINT	TRADITIONAL NAME	FUNCTION
LI 4	*Joining Valley*	Source Point. Relieves nasal congestion, sneezing or burning eyes. Relieves skin disorders and pain.
LI 11	*Crooked Pond*	Relieves skin disorders and relieves pain.
Bl 13	*Lung Back Transporting Point*	Benefits any skin condition.
Sp 6	*Three Yin Meeting*	Helps resolve skin disorders.
Sp 9	*Yin Mound Spring*	Resolves damp related disorders of the skin.

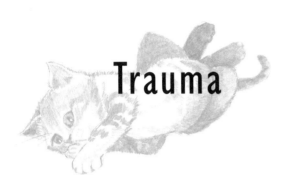

Trauma

PAIN REDUCTION

The points listed below are
emergency points and should
be used while on your way to
the clinic.

Indicators
Major physical injury
Trauma
Acute disease

Procedure
Open the Large Intestine,
Stomach, Spleen, Triple Heater
and Gall Bladder Meridians
along their entire length on
both sides of your cat.
Perform specific Point Work
on **LI 4, St 35, 39 & 44,
Sp 6, TH 23 and GB 36**

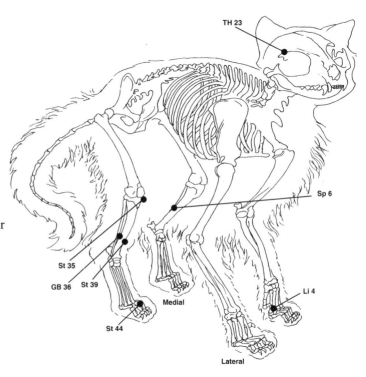

POINT	*TRADITIONAL NAME*	FUNCTION
LI 4	*Joining Valley*	Stops pain.
St 35	*Calf Nose*	Stops pain and relieves swelling.
St 39	*Lower Great Emptiness*	Helps stop pain.
St 44	*Inner Courtyard*	Stops pain and clears heat.
Sp 6	*Three Yin Meeting*	Stops pain and cools the blood.
TH 23	*Silk Bamboo Hole*	Helps stop pain.
GB 36	*Outer Mound*	Accumulation Point. Helps eliminate pain.

SHOCK

Shock, a condition characterized by collapse of the cardiovascular system, requires immediate veterinary care. The points listed below are emergency points and should be used in route to the emergency clinic.

Indicators
Major physical injury, loss of blood   Loss of consciousness
Dazed behavior

Procedure
Open the Bladder, Heart, Kidney, Triple Heater & Governing Vessel Meridians. Perform specific Point Work on **Bl 7, Ht 9, Ki 1, TH 1, GV 26 and Bai Hui Point**

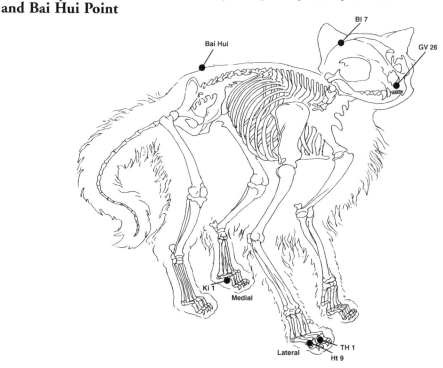

POINT	TRADITIONAL NAME	FUNCTION
Bl 7	*Reaching Heaven*	Helps retain consciousness.
Ht 9	*Lesser Yin Rushing*	Restores consciousness.
Ki 1	*Bubbling Spring*	Clears the brain and restores consciousness.
TH 1	*Gate Rush*	Restores consciousness, stops convulsions.
GV 26	*Middle of Person*	Promotes resuscitation. Regulates the balance of Yin & Yang in the body.
Bai Hui	*Hundred Meetings*	Promotes resuscitation.

143

Urinary Problems

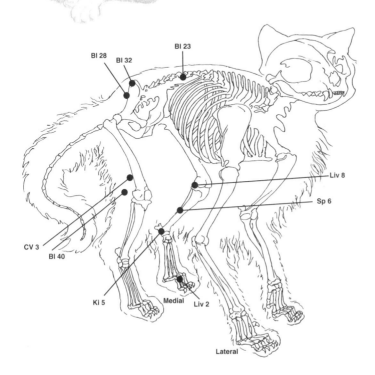

The points noted below are beneficial to the entire urinary tract. They help to strengthen the bladder and can be used to impact a variety of urinary disorders. When problems persist, consult your holistic veterinarian.

Indicators
> Difficult, strained urination
> Cystitis
> Inappropriate urination
> Frequent urination
>   or incontinence
> Blood in urine

Procedure
> Open the Bladder, Conception Vessel, Spleen, Liver and Kidney Meridians. Perform Point Work on **Bl 23, 28, 32 & 40, CV 3, Sp 6, Liv 2 & 8 and Ki 5**

POINT	TRADITIONAL NAME	FUNCTION
Bl 23	*Kidney Back Transporting Point*	A main point for strengthening the kidneys. Nourishes Kidney Essence.
Bl 28	*Bladder Back Transporting Point*	Regulates the bladder, stops pain and eliminates stagnation.
Bl 32	*Second Crevice*	Tonifies and strengthens the kidneys.
Bl 40	*Supporting Middle*	Removes obstructions from the meridian. Reduces burning urination.
CV 3	*Middle Extremity*	Alarm Point of the bladder. Promotes the Bladder function of Chi transformation. Regulates the urinary system, benefits urination.
Liv 2	*Temporary In-Between*	Source Point. Clears liver fire. Helps relieve cystitis and urethritis.
Liv 8	*Spring and Bend*	Relieves urinary burning and retention.
Ki 5	*Water Spring*	Accumulation Point. Aids urination.

Note: Conception Vessel points are located on the ventral midline of your cat.

Behavior Issues

Cats will be cats no matter what. We love them the way they are, but problems arise when cats experience stress. Depending on the cat, a stressful situation may be anything from moving a chair in your living room to moving to a new house. Cats in shelters must stoically endure highly stressful experiences. Abused and neglected cats are often fearful and sad.

Left to their own feline world, their behavior is fine. When we bring them into our homes, they have to modify their natural behavior. As discussed in Chapter One, cats have needs that do not necessarily fit into tidy, easy-to-manage packages. Living in our world can be very stressful for them. Stress can manifest as behaviors not necessarily desirable or healthy for them. The following treatment plans address some of the more common behavior difficulties.

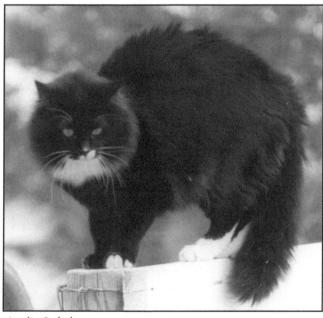

Amelia Soderberg

AGGRESSION

Indicators

Extreme domination, initiating fights   Excessive biting or scratching
Fear/Apprehension reactions   Spraying

Procedure

Open the Stomach, Heart, Kidney, Pericardium, Gall Bladder and
Governing Vessel Meridians.
Perform Point Work on **St 40, Ht 7, Pe 5, Ki 9, GB 13 and GV 11 & 24**

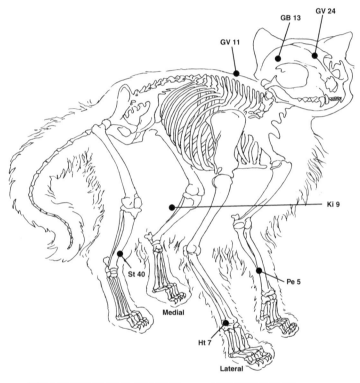

POINT	*TRADITIONAL NAME*	FUNCTION
St 40	*Abundant Bulge*	Calms and clears the mind.
Ht 7	*Mind Door*	Calms the mind, nourishes heart blood.
Pe 5	*Intermediary*	Regulates Heart Chi, relieves mental agitation.
Ki 9	*Guest Building*	Excellent calming effects, strengthens Kidney Yin.
GB 13	*Mind Root*	Calms the mind, relieves worry and jealousy.
GV 11	*Mind Way*	Calms the mind. Relieves anxiety.
GV 24	*Mind Courtyard*	Use for severe anxiety and fear.

146

ANXIETY REACTIONS

Indicators

Obsessive behaviors   Excessive meowing
Compulsive grooming   Inappropriate urination/defacation

Procedure

Open the Bladder, Heart, Pericardium and Governing Vessel Meridians.
Perform specific Point Work on **Bl 10 & 15, Ht 7, Pe 6 & 7, GV 11 and Yin Tang Point**

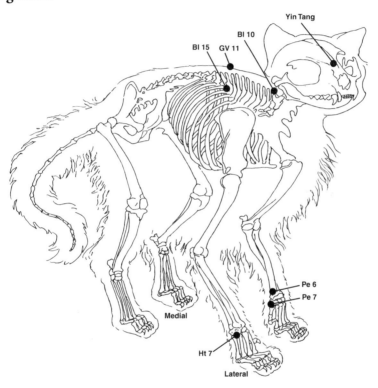

POINT	TRADITIONAL NAME	FUNCTION
Bl 10	Heavenly Pillar	Relieves stress and improves concentration.
Bl 15	Heart Back Transporting Point	Calms the mind, relieves anxiety, stimulates the brain.
Ht 7	Mind Door	Calms the mind, nourishes heart blood.
Pe 6	Inner Gate	Connecting Point. Powerful calming action on the mind.
Pe 7	Great Hill	Source & Sedation Point. Relieves great anxiety and mental restlessness.
GV 11	Mind Way	Calms the mind, relieves anxiety.
Yin Tang		Relieves anxiety.

FEAR

Indicators

Decreased appetite Excessive timidity or overly defensive
Inappropriate biting and clawing Hiding in small areas

Procedure

Open the Small Intestine, Pericardium, Gall Bladder, Liver, Conception and Governing Vessel Meridians.

Perform specific Point Work on **SI 7, Pe 3, GB 44, Liv 3, CV 15 and GV 24**

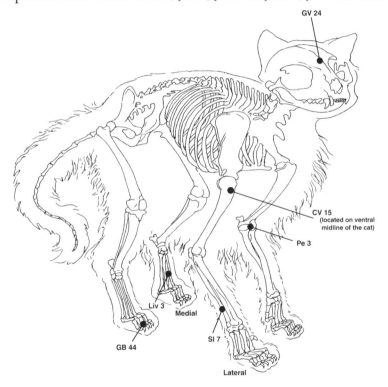

POINT	*TRADITIONAL NAME*	FUNCTION
SI 7	*Branch to the Heart*	Calms the mind in severe fear or anxiety.
Pe 3	*Middle Islet*	Lifts the mind from fear or depression.
GB 44	*Orifice Yin*	Calms the mind, helps restores confidence.
Liv 3	*Bigger Rushing*	Calms the mind, helps relieve anger.
CV 15	*Dove Tail*	Relieves fear, emotional upsets or obsessions.
GV 24	*Mind Courtyard*	Calms the mind, relieves severe fears and anxiety.

NOTE: Conception Vessel points are located on the ventral midline of your cat.

148

GRIEF/SADNESS

Indicators

Refusal to eat	Unresponsive and withdrawn
Refusal to play	Lethargic disposition

Procedure

Open the Lung, Bladder, Stomach, Heart, Gall Bladder and Governing Vessel Meridians.

Perform specific Point Work on **Lu 7, Bl 23, St 41, Ht 8, GB 12 and GV 14**

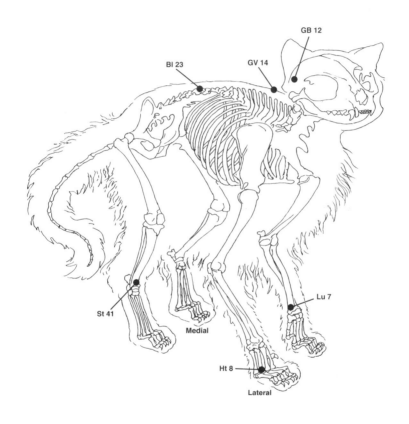

POINT	*TRADITIONAL NAME*	FUNCTION
Lu 7	*Broken Sequence*	Relieves sadness, grief and worry.
Bl 23	*Kidney Back Transporting Point*	Stimulates the spirit of initiative and lifts sadness.
St 41	*Dispersing Stream*	Clears and brightens the mind.
Ht 8	*Lesser Yin Mansion*	Sedation Point. Calms the mind.
GB 12	*Whole Bone*	Calms the mind, relieves sadness.
GV 14	*Great Palace*	Calms the mind and clears the spirit.

MENTAL CLARITY AND FOCUS

Indicators

Short attention span or inattention   Forgetfulness
Easily distracted

Procedure

Open the Bladder, Small Intestine, Gall Bladder, and Conception Vessel Meridians. Perform specific Point Work on **Bl 10 & 64, SI 3, GB 20 and CV 17**

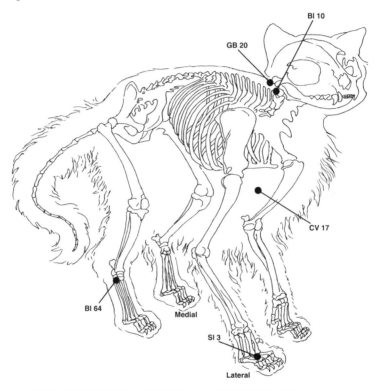

POINT	TRADITIONAL NAME	FUNCTION
Bl 10	*Heavenly Pillar*	Relieves stress and unclear thinking. Enhances concentration.
Bl 64	*Capital Bone*	Calms the mind, clears the brain, promotes clarity.
SI 3	*Back Stream*	Helps gain clarity of mind.
GB 20	*Wind Pond*	Gathers essence to the head, clears and calms the mind.
CV 17	*Middle of Chest*	Aids concentration, relieves nervousness and supports clear thinking.

Note: Conception Vessel points are located on the ventral midline of your cat.

chapter seven
Acupressure Maintenance Treatment

Some of my favorite people are cats. Every cat I have ever met has a distinct personality. Have you ever met two cats that are exactly alike? Some are too sophisticated to be bothered with playing with humans. Others can't get enough human attention. Some live to hunt while others live to sleep on the couch. All cats, however, have two attributes in common: they know what they want and when they want it. As feline members of the family, they also know they deserve to have their every whim fulfilled by the two-legged members of the family.

Once cats become accustomed to intentional touch, they thoroughly enjoy it. Jazz, a little calico, is very demanding about her twice-a-week acupressure treatments from her human. If the end of the weekend comes and her caregiver has been too busy to sit down on the couch and perform a session, Jazz lets her know, in no uncertain terms, it is time for acupressure.

In a cat's eye, all things belong to cats.
—English proverb

Terrence, an easy-going, elderly Balinese, has never enjoyed being brushed. The older he gets, the harder it is for him to keep up with his long coat. His caregiver was starting to have daily battles with him over his much-needed grooming. Terrence's human decided to give him

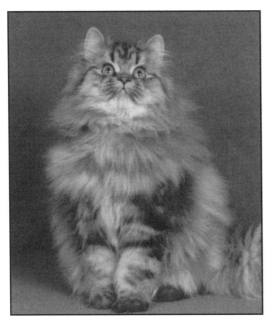

an acupressure treatment before a gentle brushing. The acupressure treatment plan includes calming acupoints such as the Yin Tang point to relieve anxiety, Heart 7 (Ht 7) to calm the mind, Governing Vessel 11 (GV 11) for calming, and Bladder 10 (Bl 10) for reducing stress.

Terrence is back being his gentle, easy-going self. He jumps up into his human's lap to have his acupressure treatment, then falls asleep while being brushed. He has come to expect an acupressure treatment and brushing two-to-three times a week.

Ongoing acupressure treatments are as invaluable for a happy, healthy cat as they are for an unhappy, sick, or injured cat. Besides, this is your opportunity to have "quality time" with your fuzzy friend. Consistently pick an evening, or some other break time during the week to spend together. Take a few minutes to relax, take deep breaths, and enjoy a playful or soothing time together before beginning your planned treatment.

Offering your healthy cat an acupressure maintenance treatment ensures that Chi energy flows freely through his entire body. Performing regularly scheduled treatments has been shown to increase mental focus and enhance physical comfort. The sensory experience combined with receiving personal attention from you–his most treasured human–is reason enough to work with your cat on a regular basis. These maintenance treatments help maintain your cat's:

- Balanced meridian system
- Vital immune system
- Well-lubricated joints
- Strong, supple muscles
- Overall sense of well-being
- Good level of energy

Stress reduction is especially key for cats that participate in shows. A show can feel like a threatening environment. Acupressure allows your cat's body and mind to relax, diminishing stress-related behaviors, plus, your consistent caring and contact helps build his self-confidence.

Through weekly repetition, you learn how your cat's energy feels and how your cat reacts to treatments when he is healthy. By gliding your hands over the meridians, you gain an awareness of how your cat's energy feels when his meridians are balanced. This knowledge of his body will alert you to any changes, giving you the advantage of addressing any sensitive areas or discomforts before they become serious blocks and manifest as a physical disease.

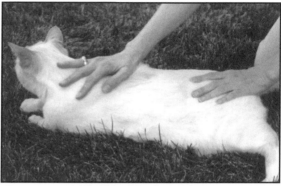
Open your cat's Bladdder Meridian to become aware of his energy.

It is very encouraging to perform maintenance treatments and see how much you contribute to your cat's well-being. His general health usually improves with only one treatment a week. These weekly acupressure treatments are good for preventive care. For instance, if your kitten is at risk for Feline Infectious Peritonitis (FIP), (a virus that is contracted by breathing or eating and spreads through cat populations in close quarters such as catteries or animal shelters), a twice-weekly Immune Strengthening treatment would be ideal to start at about six weeks old once the kitten is weaned. The kitten is protected by the mother's antibodies while nursing, but will have to build his own immune defenses after weaning.

'Oh, you wicked, wicked little thing!' cried Alice, catching up the kitten, and giving it a little kiss to make it understand that it was a disgrace. "Really, Dinah ought to have taught better manners! You ought, Dinah, you know you ought!" she added, looking reproachfully at the old cat and speaking in as cross a voice as she could manage

-Lewis Carroll,
Through the Looking-Glass

153

The maintenance treatment is similar to the treatment discussed in Chapter Three, Feline Acupressure Treatment. Be sure to work in a physical setting that is familiar and comfortable for both you and your cat. If you are traveling to a show or competition, look for an environment that has some of the same spatial features as the feeling of home. Very importantly, clear your mind of the day's activities and focus on your cat's needs. Formulate and communicate your healing intent to your cat.

Treatment Log

Recording your treatments in a Treatment Log is a valuable addition to your treatment process. Your Treatment Log book can become a useful tool for assessing your cat's wellness and becoming aware of any seasonal changes in his health, changes in mood, changes in food consumption, or changes in physical activity. In addition, the Treatment Log provides information for your veterinarian, if the need arises. During each treatment, add comments regarding your cat's current condition, such as:

- Reaction or sensitivity to a specific point
- Areas that are particularly warm or cool
- Overall muscle tone
- Physical status
- Coat condition
- Mental focus
- General responsiveness and attitude.

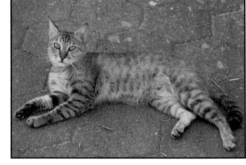

Haifa, Israel

Record your observations in the Treatment Log so you will have an ongoing record of your cat's reactions, changes, and progress. Specify the date, time of day, physical location, and description of the reaction as well as the phase of the treatment in which the reaction occurred. For example:

2/22/00 - 2:00 P.M. -
Opening: Sophie's neck feels stiff and tense.
Point Work: muscle spasms in the lower mid-neck area, lasting about 4 seconds. Reaction was followed by several long yawns and licking her front paws. Worked Bl 20, 23, 24, & 40, GB 29, and Bai Hui Point
Closing: no muscle spasms, back felt relaxed. Sophie seems calmer.

Acupressure Treatment Log

Record the meridians and acupoints you select along with your observations of your cat during each acupressure treatment.

Cat's name: _____ **Date:** _____ **Time:** _____

Pre-treatment observations: _____

_____

_____

Acupressure treatment observations: _____

_____

Opening: _____

_____

Point Work: _____

_____

Closing: _____

_____

Post-treatment observations: _____

_____

_____

Maintenance Treatment Procedure

Please refer to Chapter Three, Feline Acupressure Treatment, for a description of the Opening technique.

Opening

Open the meridians on the front of your cat by stroking down his neck, over his shoulder and down the inside and outside of his front legs. Repeat this procedure on the opposite side of your cat.

Open the meridians on your cat's abdomen and back by stroking along his back and the side of his abdomen and flank, then stroke down the inside and outside of his hind legs. Repeat this procedure on the opposite side of your cat.

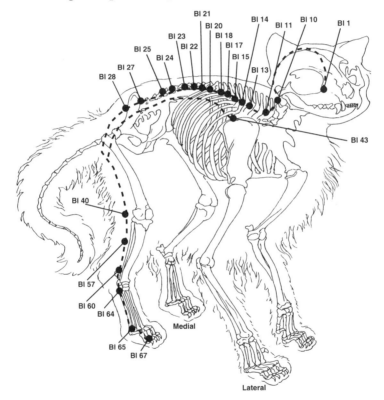

Point Work

Work the Bladder meridian on both sides of your cat's body. The Association Points for each of the organ systems are located along the Bladder meridian. These points help balance your cat's Chi energy throughout his body.

Note reactions and sensitivity to a particular point or area of your cat's body. Feel for areas of heat or coolness, protrusion or depression, sponginess or densefness, to determine if the points are excessive or deficient of Chi. If you find specific Association Points that are excessive or deficient in Chi, additional Point

EXCESS ACUPOINTS	DEFICIENT ACUPOINTS
Protruding	Depressed
Warm	Cool or Cold
Painful or Sensitive	Vacant or Empty
Hard or Dense	Soft or Spongy
Acute	Chronic

Work is needed along the associated organ meridian. Generally, when a point is cool and depressed, it needs tonification. If it feels warm and protrudes, sedate the point. Record your observations in your Treatment Log and monitor your cat's condition during your next maintenance treatment.

Check all Ting Points for excessive and deficient characteristics. If you find an imbalance in one or more of these points, sedate or tonify each point in response to what the point evinces. Some practitioners find that balancing only the Ting Points is sufficient for treating many conditions.

If your cat does not exhibit excessive or deficient areas or reactive points that indicate a disharmony, enjoy his good health and move to Closing. If your cat is not well or seems to be experiencing stress, refer to Chapter 6, Acupressure Treatments for Specific Conditions. Create a treatment plan including specific acupoints that directly relate to the type of attention your cat needs.

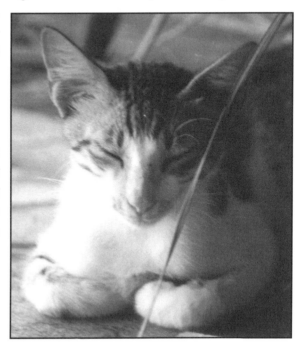

Closing

To Close work from front to rear, top to bottom by gliding your hand over the Bladder meridian. Refer to Chapter 3, Feline Acupressure Treatment, for a detailed description of the Closing techniques.

Cats give us so many gifts. They have served as mousers, sweet companions, and playmates. They have provided great moments of amusement, deep feelings of love and tender consolation. Cats have been a rich source of creative inspiration and imagery for some of the finest artists, poets, novelists, composers, cinematographers...those who contribute to our rich culture. What would Carl Sandburg's diminutive poem, "Fog," be like without "little cat feet?"

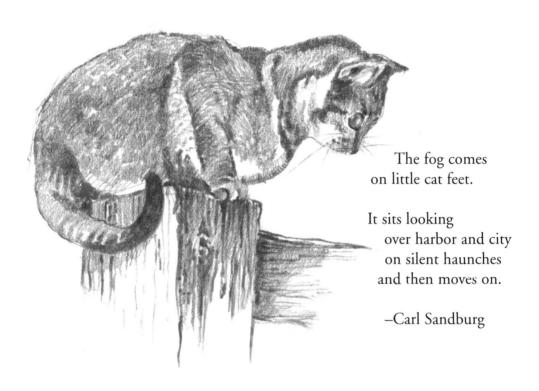

The fog comes
on little cat feet.

It sits looking
    over harbor and city
    on silent haunches
    and then moves on.

–Carl Sandburg

For most of us, our feline friends offer a respite from the daily expectations of work, family demands and all the hustle and bustle of our lives. Spend your "cat time" returning the favors your cat brings just by being your cat. Acupressure gives you another way to enjoy each other's company while adding the pleasure of knowing you are both healing.

GLOSSARY

ACCUMULATION POINTS Specific acupressure points located on a meridian where the Chi accumulates. Used primarily for acute conditions, especially if pain is present.

ACUPOINTS Specific points located on a meridian where the Chi energy flows close to the surface of the body. Stimulation, tonification, sedation and other techniques can be employed to manipulate the Chi energy of the body at these locations.

ACUPRESSURE An ancient healing art that moves and balances Chi energy by use of pressure applied at specific acupoints along the meridian system. Used to release muscular pain, tension, to increase circulation and treat a variety of ailments and conditions by balancing life force energy.

ACUPUNCTURE The manipulation of Chi energy by use of needle insertions at specific acupoints along the meridian system. Used to release muscular pain, tension, to increase circulation and treat a variety of ailments and conditions by balancing life force energy.

ACUTE A condition having a short and relatively sudden course, not long term.

ALARM POINTS Used as indicators of organ and meridian problems. Tenderness at an Alarm Point gives the practitioner an indication of meridian blockage or organ involvement. Alarm Points are used in conjunction with the Association Points.

ANTIINFLAMMATORY An agent that relieves inflammation of the tissues.

ANTIOXIDANT A substance that inhibits the metabolic reactions promoted by oxygen.

ASPIRIN POINT An acupoint located on the Bladder meridian, Bl 60, known for its ability to reduce pain throughout the body.

ASSOCIATED MERIDIANS A pair of Yin and Yang meridians. Each of the twelve major meridians has an associated meridian partner, making a total of six paired meridians. Point Work on either of the paired meridians serves to balance the energy flow of the other.

ASSOCIATION POINTS Specific points located along the first channel of the Bladder meridian. Each of the twelve major meridians has a unique Association Point. Association Points can indicate a blockage in the corresponding meridian and are used in conjunction with the Alarm Points to help identify the level of organ involvement.

ATROPHY Decrease in size of muscle or organ resulting from lack of use or disease.

AUTOIMMUNE DISEASE A condition in which the white blood cells destroy the tissues of the organism that created them.

AXIAL SKELETON The part of the skeleton consisting of the spinal column and skull.

BELLY The abdomen or ventral region of the body from the xiphoid cartilage of the sternum to the edge of the pelvis.

BICEPS FEMORIS The two headed muscle located in the upper hind leg.

BIOKINETICS The study of the movement of animals.

BLADDER MERIDIAN One of the twelve major meridians. It is a Yang meridian and is paired with the Kidney meridian, a Yin energy meridian. The Association Points are located on the Bladder meridian.

BREASTBONE The ventral bone to which the ribs attach, sternum or breast plate.

BURSA A sac located under a tendon or over a bony prominence filled with heavy fluid. Theses sacs reduce friction.

CARPAL JOINT The wrist or fore pastern. A complex joint between the distal ends of the radius and ulna and the metacarpal bones.

CARTILAGE The elastic material that covers the articular surfaces of joints.

CHANNEL CHI The aspect of Chi that flows through the meridian or channel system. It is the aspect of Chi that is most available for adjustment or influence by acupressure or acupuncture.

CHEST The external anatomical region of the ribs or thorax.

CHI ENERGY Life force energy which is present in all of nature. There are a variety of "types" of Chi, defined by location and function.

CHRONIC A condition that persists for a long time with little change or improvement.

CLOSING The third phase of an acupressure treatment. The Closing serves to connect the energy flow between the points stimulated during the treatment. It also helps repattern cellular memory and relieve chronic pain.

CLOSING TECHNIQUES Specific techniques used by the acupressure practitioner to complete the Closing phase of an acupressure treatment. Techniques include smooth hand and cupped hand.

COCCYGEAL The terminal vertebrae of the spinal column, pertaining to the tail.

COLLATERAL LIGAMENTS The fibrous bands located on either side of a joint that serve to stabilize the joint and hold the bones in normal apposition to each other.

COMMAND POINT Also known as "Element" points. Command Points are employed when referencing the Five-Element Theory to either tonify or sedate, based on the Control and Creation Cycle.

CONCEPTION VESSEL One of the eight Extraordinary Vessels. A Yin vessel passing unilaterally along the ventral midline.

CONNECTING POINTS These points connect the Yin and Yang energies of the sister meridians. These points help resolve blockages between the sister meridians. Also known as "Luo" Points.

CONTROL CYCLE The sequence of the Five-Element Theory in which each element controls another and is itself controlled by another element. This sequence helps ensure that a balance is maintained among the five elements.

CREATION CYCLE The sequence of the Five-Element Theory in which each element creates another and is itself created by another element. This sequence helps ensure that a balance is maintained among the five elements.

DEFICIENCY A condition of insufficiency or too little of something. In TCM a deficiency often refers to insufficient energy, indicating the need to improve or increase energy in that area.

DEWCLAW The inside toe on a cat's leg corresponding to the human thumb. It is a vestigial digit.

DIGITS The toes of a cat.

DISTAL POINTS Acupressure points located a distance from the area they benefit.

EDEMA The accumulation of abnormally large amounts of fluid between the cells in the tissues.

ELBOW The hinge joint connecting the humerus to the radius and ulna.

ESTROUS The entire reproductive cycle of the cat. Regularly occurring periods during which the female is sexually active and receptive.

EXCESS A condition of surplus or too much of something.. In TCM an excess often refers to an over-abundance of energy, indicating the need to decrease or disperse the energy in that area.

EXTENSOR The muscles that extend a joint.

EXTRAORDINARY VESSELS Eight Vessels which act as reservoirs of energy for the major meridians. They absorb energy from the major meridians or transfer energy to the major meridians as needed.

FEMUR The large bone that extends down from the coxofemoral joint of the pelvis to the stifle.

FIBULA The smaller of the two bones of the lower hind leg that extend from the stifle to the hock.

FOOD CHI Life force energy (Chi) obtained from food.

FOREARM The lower foreleg, between the elbow and carpus.

FOREPASTERN The anatomical region between the carpus and the toes.

FOREPAW The front foot.

FU ORGANS The six Yang organs, also referred to as the hollow organs.

GALL BLADDER MERIDIAN One of the twelve major meridians. It is a Yang meridian and is paired with the Liver meridian, a Yin energy meridian.

GASTROINTESTINAL Pertaining to the stomach and intestines. It can refer to the entire digestive tract.

GLUTEAL MUSCLES The muscle group over the croup and pelvis.

GOVERNING VESSEL One of the Eight Extraordinary Vessels. This is a Yang vessel that runs unilaterally along the dorsal midline.

HAMSTRING The tendon of the biceps femoris muscle of the hind leg.

HAUNCH The region of the hips and buttocks.

HEART MERIDIAN One of the twelve major meridians. It is a Yin meridian and is paired with the Small Intestine meridian, a Yang energy meridian.

HINDQUARTERS The anatomical body area located behind the flanks and includes the pelvis, thighs and hocks.

HIP JOINT The joint between the femur and the pelvis.

HIP SOCKET The pelvic cavity into which fits the head of the femur and with which it articulates.

HOCK The ankle joint of quadrupeds. The tarsus or joint between the stifle and pastern.

HUMERUS The upper arm bone, that which extends from the shoulder to the elbow.

ILIUM The pelvic bone on which the hip socket is located. It connects to the sacral vertebrae at the sacroiliac junction.

INFLUENTIAL POINTS Points which affect a particular functional system.

INTERVERTEBRAL DISK The cushioning structure located between the bodies of adjacent vertebrae.

JING The life essence, or material aspect of Chi, a fundamental substance.

KIDNEY MERIDIAN One of the twelve major meridians. It is a Yin meridian and is paired with the Bladder meridian,
a Yang energy meridian.

KNEE The stifle joint.

KNEECAP The patella. A sesmoid bone located on the anterior surface of the stifle joint.

KNUCKLE The metacarpal or metatarsal joint. The dorsal surface of any foot joint.

LAME An irregularity or impairment of the function of locomotion or gaits.

LARGE INTESTINE MERIDIAN One of the twelve major meridians. It is a Yang meridian and is paired with the Lung meridian, a Yin energy meridian.

LATERAL Toward the outside of the body.

LIGAMENTS Connective tissue that binds joints together and connects bones and cartilage.

LIVER MERIDIAN One of the twelve major meridians. It is a Yin meridian and is paired with the Gall Bladder meridian, a Yang energy meridian.

LOCAL POINTS Acupressure points located in the area they benefit.

LOIN The anatomical area of the back between the last rib and the pelvis.

LUMBAR Pertaining to the loins, the part of the back between the thorax and pelvis.

LUMBOSACRAL JOINT Located at the top of the croup, it rotates the hindquarters and pelvis forward under the body.

LUNG CHI Life energy (Chi) which is extracted from the air.

LUNG MERIDIAN One of the twelve major meridians. It is a Yin meridian and is paired with the Large Intestine meridian, a Yang energy meridian.

MASTER POINT Acupoints which powerfully affect a regional area of the body. There are six Master Points.

MEDIAL Toward the center of the body.

MERIDIAN BLOCKAGE A condition which impedes the smooth, even and balanced flow of Chi energy throughout the meridian system.

MERIDIAN SYSTEM The network of invisible but real channels through which the Chi (life force) energy flows throughout the body. These channels are connected and influence each other.

MERIDIANS Individual channels that are part of a network through which Chi energy flows throughout the body. There are twelve major meridians in all animals.

METACARPUS The bones leading from the carpus or wrist to the toes.

METATARSUS The bones leading from the tarsus or hock to the toes.

OCCIPITAL CREST The highest point of the head.

OPENING The first phase of an acupressure treatment. The Opening introduces "structured" touch to the animal. The Opening also affords the practitioner the opportunity to identify areas of the body which may need Point Work.

ORIGINAL CHI The fixed amount of Chi given at conception. Also known as Source Chi.

PALPATION Feeling or perceiving by the sense of touch.

PASTERN The region of the metatarsus extending from the hock to the foot in the hind leg and the metacarpal area of the foreleg.

PATELLA Kneecap. A large sesamoid bone at the femorotibial joint.

PAW Any of the cat's four feet.

PECTORAL Pertaining to the chest or breast area.

PELVIC LIMB Either hind leg.

PELVIS The bony girdle comprised of the Ilium, ischium and pubis.

PERICARDIUM MERIDIAN One of the twelve major meridians. It is a Yin meridian and is paired with the Triple Heater meridian, a Yang energy meridian.

POINT OF ELBOW The olecanon process of the ulna bone.

POINT OF HOCK The summit of the calcaneus.

POINT OF SHOULDER The junction of the humerus and the shoulder blade.

POINT WORK The stimulation of acupoints located along the meridian system.

POINT WORK TECHNIQUES The procedures used to stimulate points. There are several techniques a practitioner may use, each of which has a unique quality.

PROTECTIVE CHI The Chi that protects the body from harmful external forces.

PROXIMAL Nearer to or toward the center, or midline, of the body.

RADIUS One of the two bones of the forearm which extends from the elbow to the carpus.

REAR PASTERN The anatomical area between the hock and the foot.

SEDATE To disperse or decrease.

SEDATION POINT Points which subdue an excess of energy within the meridian flow.

SCAPULA The shoulder blade.

SHEN Represents the "spirit" aspect of Chi energy.

SHOCK A condition of acute peripheral circulatory failure due to derangement of circulatory control or loss of circulating fluid.

SKELETON The bony framework of the body.

SMALL INTESTINE MERIDIAN One of the twelve major meridians. It is a Yang meridian and is paired with the Heart meridian, a Yin energy meridian.

SOURCE POINTS A specific point directly connected to each of the twelve major meridians. The Source Point can either sedate or tonify, depending upon the need of the meridian at the time of stimulation.

SPINOUS PROCESSES The upward projections of each vertebrae.

SPLEEN MERIDIAN One of the twelve major meridians. It is a Yin meridian and is paired with the Stomach meridian, a Yang energy meridian.

STIFLE The "knee" on the hind leg of the cat.

STOMACH MERIDIAN One of the twelve major meridians. It is a Yang meridian and is paired with the Spleen, a Yin energy meridian.

TARSUS The hock or ankle.

TENDONS Tissue that connects muscle to bone, they are strong and inelastic.

THIGH The region of hind leg that lies above the stifle and below the hip.

THORACIC VERTEBRAE The thirteen bones that form the top of the rib cage.

TIBIA The lower leg bone extending from the stifle to the tarsus.

TING POINT Located at the cat's front and hind legs. These points are either the beginning or ending of the meridians and there is one Ting Point for each meridian. Used to balance the energy of the meridian and for other specific conditions.

TONIFICATION POINTS A specific acupoint located on each of twelve major meridians. Stimulation of these points tonifies or adds energy to that meridian.

TONIFY To increase or strengthen.

TRIPLE HEATER One of the twelve major meridians. It is a Yang meridian and is paired with the Pericardium meridian, a Yin energy meridian.

ULNA A bone of the foreleg which extends from the elbow joint to the carpus.

UPPER ARM The anatomical area between the elbow and the shoulder.

VASCULAR SYSTEM Blood vessel network of the body.

WRIST The complex joint between the radius and ulna and the metacarpals.

YANG Part of the Yin/Yang duality. Some attributes associated with Yang include: warmth, outer, sunny side, movement, acute, light, male.

YIN Part of the Yin/Yang duality. Some attributes associated with Yin include: cold, inner, shady side, substance, chronic, dark, female.

ZANG The six Yin organs, also referred to as the solid organs.

BIBLIOGRAPHY

Altman, Sheldon, DVM. *An Introduction to Acupuncture for Animals.* Chen's Corporation, Monterey Park, CA. 1981.

Beinfield, Harriet, L.Ac. & Korngold, Efrem, L. Ac., OMD. *Between Heaven and Earth, A Guide to Chinese Medicine.* Ballentine Books, New York, NY. 1991.

Bicks, Jane, DVM. *Revolution in Cat Nutrition,* Rawson Associates, New York, 1986.

Bicks, Jane, DVM. *Dr. Jane's Thirty Days to a Healthier, Happier Cat,* Berkeley Publishing, NY, 1997.

Birch, Stephen and Matsumoto, Kiiko, *Five Elements and Ten Stems.* Paradigm Publications, Brookline, MA 1983.

Connelly, Dianne, M., Ph.D., M. Ac. *Traditional Acupuncture: The Law of the Five Elements.* The Centre for Traditional Acupuncture, Columbia, MD. 1989.

Fogle, Bruce, Dr. *Natural Cat Care.* D K Publishing, CO, New York, NY 1999.

International Veterinary Acupuncture Society, The Chinese Acupuncture, 5,000 Year Old Oriental Art of Healing.

Lazarus, Pat. *Keep Your Cat Healthy the Natural Way.* The Ballantine Publishing Group, New York, NY 1983.

Maciocia, Giovanni, CaC. *The Foundations of Chinese Medicine, A Comprehensive Text for Acupuncturists and Herbalists.* Churchill Livingstone. New York, NY 1989.

Manning, Clark A. and Vanrenen, Louis J. *Bioenergetic Medicines East and West Acupuncture and Homeopathy.* North Atlantic Books, Berkeley, CA 1988.

Milani, Myrna M, DVM. *The Body Language and Emotion of Cats.* William Morrow Co, NY 1987.

Puotinen, C.J. *The Encyclopedia of Natural Pet Care.* Keats Publishing, Inc, New Canaan, CT 1998.

Ross, Jeremy. *Acupuncture Point Combinations, The Key to Clinical Success.* Churchill Livingstone, New York, NY 1998.

Schwartz, Cheryl, DVM. *Four Paws Five Directions, A Guide to Chinese Medicine for Cats and Dogs.* Celestial Arts, Berkeley, CA, 1996.

Thomas, Elizabeth Marshall, *The Tribe of Tiger.* Simon & Schuster, New York, NY 1994.

Zidonis, Nancy A, Snow, Amy and Soderberg, Marie K. *Equine Acupressure: A Working Manual.* Tallgrass Publishers, LLC, Denver, CO 1998.

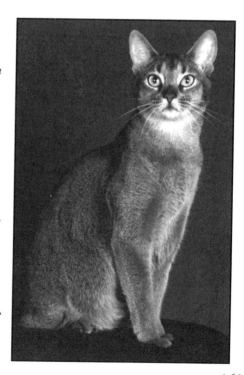

TALLGRASS TRAINING PROGRAMS

Tallgrass offers highly interactive training programs for people committed to promoting the natural health, well-being and spirit of animals.

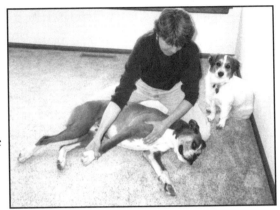

- Introductory: Acupressure concepts and theory, methods of observation, acupoint and meridian system hands on experience.
- Intermediate: Acupressure theory and meridian system review, hands- on Point Work for specific conditions, in-depth work with the Five Phases of Transformation and other complementary healing modalities.

For further information or to host a clinic, contact Tallgrass Training. Call 888.841.7211, fax 303.777.8877, or visit our website at www.tallgrasspublishers.com.

TALLGRASS PUBLISHERS' SIGNATURE ARTIST: CARLA STROH

Animal Portraiture is Carla Stroh's passion. She has brought her award winning talent and intuitive senses to hundreds of animal portraits for over twenty years. For the past ten years, Carla has been the exclusive illustrator of Tallgrass Publisher's books on animal acupressure. Our readers have commented how much they appreciate her work.

Now, we can offer Carla's artistic gifts to you. Send us a photograph of your cat, dog, horse, or any favorite animal, and Carla can create a portrait. Select the medium; she works in graphite, pastels, pen and ink, watercolor, and acrylic.

Capture the image and vitality of your loving animals in a permanent piece of art. Send us your photograph; note the choice of medium and Carla will get back to you with a cost estimate. You will enjoy the having a painting or drawing your pet for the rest of your life.

Send photographs to: Tallgrass Publishers, PO Box 101747, Denver, CO 80210, or call for further information, 303.777.4744.

164

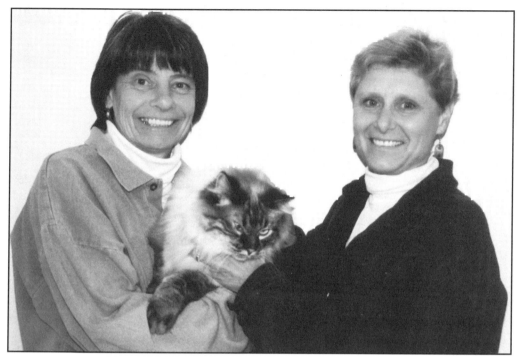

Photo: Jan Jones

Profiles

Acu-Cat: A Guide to Feline Acupressure is the collaborative effort of Nancy Zidonis and Amy Snow. Each has contributed their talents, skills and knowledge with the intent of making acupressure accessible for every one to enjoy. In the past two years, Nancy and Amy have published *Equine Acupressure: A Working Manual* and *The Well-Connected Dog: A Guide to Canine Acupressure*.

Over the past 15 years, Nancy Zidonis has co-authored other acupressure texts, and developed equine, canine and feline meridian charts as well as acupressure training programs. She teaches acupressure throughout the United States and Europe and is a founding board member of The International Alliance of Animal Therapy and Healing (IAATH). As a child in rural Ohio, Nancy thoroughly enjoyed and respected the integrity of the animals in her life. Writing and teaching acupressure is her on-going contribution.

Amy Snow has combined her professional publications background and experience in the healing arts with her love of all animals in co-authoring this book. When growing up in New York City she longed for a time and place to devote her life to the care and welfare of gentle animals. Teaching acupressure allows her the opportunity to offer people and animals a meaningful way to care for each other.

Nancy and Amy are currently working on a series of human acupressure books that will be available in the fall of 2000. Watch for *Acu-Rider, Acu-Golfer* and *Acu-Hiker/Runner*.

order form

FELINE
Acu-Cat: A Guide to Feline Acupressure. (ISBN 0-9645982-5-6) Item # 0001 / Unit Price $23.95
Feline Meridian Chart. 12 x 18 color, laminated chart. Item # 9805 / Unit Price $16.00

CANINE
The Well-Connected Dog: A Guide to Canine Acupressure. (ISBN 0-9645982-4-8) Item # 9905
Unit Price $25.95
Canine Meridian Chart. 12 x 18 color, laminated chart. Item # 9806 / Unit Price $16.00

EQUINE
Equine Acupressure, A Working Manual. (ISBN 0-9645982-2-1) Item # 9801 / Unit Price $29.95

Equine Meridian Chart. 12x18 color, laminated chart. Item # 9802 / Unit Price $16.00

Equine Stretch Poster. 12x18 laminated poster. Item # 9803 / Unit Price $16.00

Five-Element Meridian Chart Set. Includes 4 - 12x18 color, laminated charts of meridian system:
Twelve Major Meridians, Governing and Conception Vessels, Accumulation, Alarm, Association,
Command, Connecting,Source, and Ting Points. Plus Five-Element Theory chart. Item # 9804
Unit Price $53.50 (CALL FOR DISTRIBUTOR DISCOUNTS)
New! Equine Acupressure Video. 45 minute Instructional Introductory Tape, companion to the
Equine Acupressure Book. Item #0002 / Unit Price $30.95

Ordered By:	Ship to: (If Different)
Name:	Name:
Street/POB:	Street/POB:
City/Zip:	City/Zip:

ITEM #	DESCRIPTION	QTY	UNIT PRICE	TOTAL AMT.

Shipping & Handling (Canada + $6.00)		Subtotal (USA Funds)	
1-2 Books $4.00	3-6 Books $7.00	CO Res. 3.8%	
1-3 Charts $5.00	4-6 Charts $7.00	S & H	
		TOTAL	

PAYMENT TO TALLGRASS PUBLISHERS,LLC:
❑ Check   ❑ Money Order   ❑ VISA/Master Card
VISA/MC #:   Expiration Date: Signature:

TO ORDER: FAX: 303.777.8877 e-mail tallgrasspub@earthlink.net
CALL: 888.841.7211/303.777.4744 SEND TO: Tallgrass Publishers, POB 101747, Denver, CO 80210
Website: tallgrasspublishers.com or animalacupressure.com